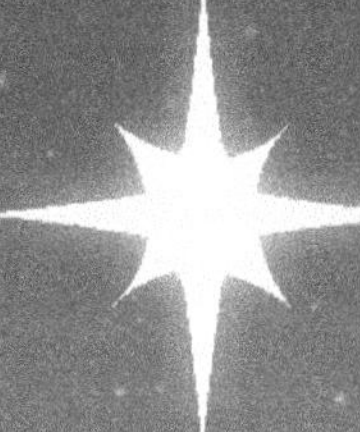

FINDING KiND

Discovering Hope *and* Purpose *while* Loving Kids *with* Invisible Neurological Differences

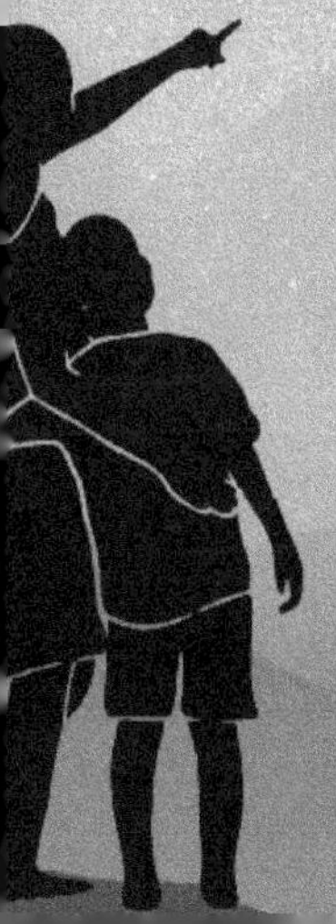

KARI A. BAKER

Foreword by Brady Baker

First Print Edition, 2024
Printed in China

Publishing Services: Jodi Cowles, Brandon Janous, and Rachael Mitchell (Blue Hat Publishing)
Cover Design: Rachael Mitchell (Blue Hat Publishing)
Interior Layout: Tim Marshall (Blue Hat Publishing)

ISBN: 978-1-962674-14-0

BLUE HAT
PUBLISHING
BOISE • KNOXVILLE • NASHVILLE • SEATTLE
WWW.BLUEHATPUBLISHING.COM

To John and Brady, for trusting me to tell our family's story, and for making me a KIND mom.

TABLE OF CONTENTS

FOREWORD

Hi, my name is Brady Baker. I am thirteen years old, and I have autism and ADHD. But neither of these things are as bad as they sound. I know you probably just want to skip ahead and see what my amazing mom has to say, but this is my side of the story. The first thing I want to say is that autism is not like a cancer trying to invade a person's mind, it's a neurologically altered perspective. I might be more interested in a person's shirt than their face or care more about a costume that a character in *Star Wars* wears than whether Vader is Luke's dad. The point I am trying to make is just because I think differently, stutter a little, and have a hard time connecting with people I don't know, from my perspective it's normal. You are the one who seems different to me.

ADHD is not what you think either. It's like that one scene at the end of *Lord of the Rings: The Return of the King* when Frodo is about to throw the evil ring into a huge volcano. But at the last second, he gains an unhealthy obsession with the ring and decides to keep it. It takes some outside intervention from Gollum ("MY PRECIOUS!!!") and Samwise to make Frodo ditch the ring, along with one of his fingers.

So, Frodo was having something resembling an ADHD moment with the ring. I don't mean the things I focus on are an evil piece of bling created by the dark lord Sauron to make him all-powerful. I mean ADHD sometimes distracts me from what other people think are important things and makes me hyperfocus on a preferred distraction.

ADHD doesn't eliminate any chance of doing well in school or in life either. For example, if you have ADHD and you love DC

Comics, you could do their marketing and have a good chance of succeeding in that! Or if you really love history class in school you could consider an academic path! For me, I love writing and movies, so I want to be an author or a film director.

I know, I know. You still want to see what my mom has to say, so this is where we part. KIND Parents, (you'll learn what KIND stands for in the book) even if your child's brain works differently, like mine, he still has a lot of things he can offer to the world. And for the kids, always know even if you have some setbacks, every human is fearfully and wonderfully made, so you can achieve greatness.

iNTRODUCTiON

I was sitting on the carpet just inside the door to my bedroom, hugging my knees close to my chest, my heart pounding and my eyes stinging from tears. Across the house, I listened to my four-year-old son Brady scream between sobs, "MOMMY!! MOMMY!! COME BACK!! MOMMY!!" I didn't respond. Repeatedly, he begged me to come to him, but I wouldn't. I sat silently, hidden from his view. I knew he couldn't get to me. He hadn't yet mastered the fine motor skills necessary to break free from the child gate that separated his side of the house from mine.

My mind ran through all the terrible things that could happen on the other side of the gate in the following moments. He could start throwing or breaking things, but I reminded myself that "things" were not important and could be replaced. I was more terrified that he would injure himself: bang his head against the wall or tile floor, run through the garage into the street, grab something sharp. The scenarios were endless and running on a loop in my brain. How could I ever forgive myself if he got hurt?

As I continued to listen to his cries, I tried to piece together the events that turned the last few minutes into a raging dumpster fire. All I could remember was telling him he had to wash his hands after going to the bathroom. When he refused, I said he couldn't watch his YouTube video until he complied. That was it, the beginning of a DEFCON 5 meltdown. Not quite *Mommie Dearest* material to me, but apparently a major infringement to Brady. In his rage, he kicked, punched, and said things that tore my heart in two.

This wasn't the first time a meltdown of this magnitude had occurred. Brady had been diagnosed with autism about a year earlier, so we weren't exactly rookies. But this one was escalating into something I was afraid would leave permanent scars on us both.

Desperate to diffuse the situation, I decided to try a new strategy the therapists affectionately called "Poker Face." Usually when Brady had a tantrum, I had one too, in a manner of speaking. I would get frustrated, order him to settle down, and even try to physically control him. My actions only added to the chaos. We learned that my behavior was feeding his response, the exact opposite of my intention. Instead, she wanted us to stop interacting with him completely until he was able to calm down. Attention was a reward for good behavior, not a response to bad behavior, according to the therapist. But she wasn't sitting next to me listening to the horror movie soundtrack down the hall.

Still, I willed myself to stay on the floor of my room and wait, praying the collateral damage—both physical and emotional—would be limited.

When I sensed a break in the outbursts, I took a deep breath and tried to use my most calm, collected voice to say, "Brady, I can't come out until you are nice to me. I can't be with you if you hurt me. When you settle down and say something kind, I will come out."

There were several seconds of silence before he finally stopped crying and muttered, "OK, Mommy. I'm hungry." Not exactly the apology I was looking for, but it would have to do. I got up, walked out of my door, and strolled back to him, forcing the muscles in my face to relax to a neutral expression. I opened the gate and went into the kitchen to make lunch like the episode never happened. Brady moved on, and I went into silent recovery mode, licking my emotional wounds and replaying the scene in my head, attempting to figure out what in the world I could have done differently.

That was almost a decade ago, and it seems like another life. As I write this book, Brady is a happy, sweet, smart, funny, courageous teenager. He still has autism, of course, and we've added ADHD and a couple of other ingredients to his neurological soup. But it is hard for me to reconcile that the screaming child in the story I just described is the same kid we know and love today.

In the middle of the long days and weeks of any challenge, forward progress can appear elusive. Changes are so gradual, so subtle, we often wonder whether we're gaining any ground at all or if all of our efforts are an exercise in futility. But time is the great illuminator, and the years have given me a new perspective. Brady's baby steps have accumulated into a giant leap ahead. He has learned to communicate, to self-regulate, and to appreciate his strengths. In the process, God gave me a new purpose: to write the book I desperately needed but couldn't find all those years ago.

When Brady was diagnosed, I found plenty of dry, technical textbooks and medical journals, but what I craved was understanding, community, and some picture of what life would be like further down the road when Brady was older. I wanted to know I wasn't alone. I wanted to peek into someone else's family for reassurance that ours wasn't some horrible anomaly. I wanted to hear stories of hope—the good, the bad, and the funny. Because trust me, if there is one thing you need in your toolbox as a parent of a neurodiverse child, it's humor. Enough time has passed to be able to chuckle at some of the debacles we had in our parenting journey and to recognize the clear blessings and provision that we experienced as Brady grew into a smart, sweet, loving, fun, faith-filled, creative young man.

So, when I had the opportunity to sell my business and walk away from a thirty-year career in the financial services industry, I did. I took my own leap. I started KIND Families, a community for anyone who loves Kids with Invisible Neurological Differences. I started blogging and speaking about our experiences, and podcasting on KIND-related topics. And I wrote the book.

You will probably notice quickly that Jesus is one of the main characters in my stories because he is the main character in my life. But if you are not someone who has found your faith yet, this book is still for you! My faith came as a beautiful result of some of the true stories I want to share with you, and I think they will resonate regardless of your beliefs.

What you will not find in this book is a platform for debate. While I will tirelessly advocate for my son, it is not my intention to discuss what causes neurodiversity in children, which therapies are good or bad, or any other hot topic that may push your buttons one way or another. I am also not a doctor, therapist, or autism expert, so please don't misconstrue anything in this book as advice for treating a child with autism.

I am just a mom who learned to recognize my control issues and planning tendencies were keeping me from embracing the beautiful life I already had. But when I finally began to trust in God's plan for me and Brady, I found my hope, and I found my purpose. My prayer is that you will too.

PART 1:

AWAKENiNG

"God is looking for those with whom He can do the impossible– what a pity that we plan only the things that we can do by ourselves."

—*A.W Tozer*

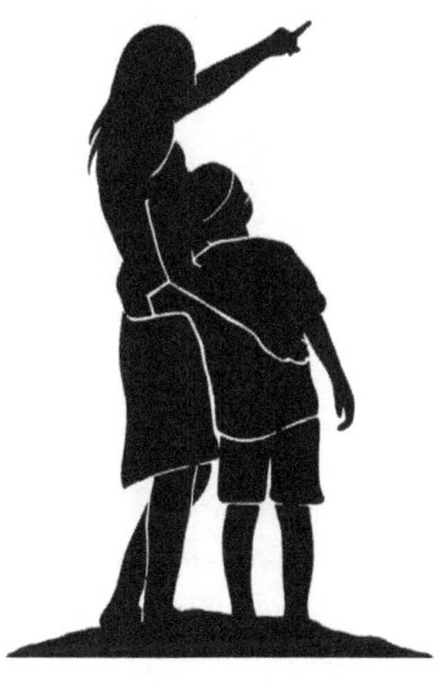

CHAPTER 1
iN THE BEGiNNiNG

I've heard lots of my friends say they always wanted to be a mom. That's true for me, but not because of a lifelong yearning to bear children. Motherhood was just part of my plan. From the time I was a little girl, I knew I wanted to have a successful career, get married, and have children, preferably in that order. The career part came easy, but I won't lie; I started getting a little nervous about the rest of it when I was still single in my early thirties.

Apparently my mother was worried too, because my Christmas present in 2004 was a subscription to a matchmaking service and a full set of pots and pans. She wanted me to find a husband and learn how to cook, not necessarily in that order. The clock was ticking, and she wasn't messing around with her chance to be a grandmother.

After a couple mediocre dates from the matchmaker, and one full blown trainwreck, I hit the jackpot. John was handsome, smart, accomplished, responsible, and always called when he said he would. We both canceled our subscription to the dating service and have been together ever since. He took a little longer to propose than I would have liked, but we finally got married when I was 37. My mom's plan worked like a charm, except for the cooking part. Never has a Christmas gift been so tragically neglected.

I am a planner by nature, and a bit of a control freak, so all those little delays leading up to pending motherhood were annoying, but bearable. Especially when I took one of those little stick tests just after my 39th birthday and passed.

I celebrated getting fat for the first time in my life and relished nine whole months of not having to suck in my tummy. When we went to a restaurant John would ask me, "What are you going to order with your French fries?" Carbs were my long-lost friends. I had missed them so much!

I had some weird complications with my pregnancy, including almost constant nausea for several months. I don't know who came up with the term morning sickness, but for me, it was an all-day affair. Brady's placenta also attached itself to the wrong place in my body, which caused me to be on major activity restrictions. I attribute his misplacement in my womb to the reason he still has a hard time putting things away where they belong.

I had an appointment to deliver Brady via C-section on February 15th, about a week before my due date. Brady was breech

and positioned so that a C-section was necessary, and frankly I was fine with that. My planner's heart loved the fact that I got to set a date and just show up to have the baby–no surprises. The doctor tried to schedule it for the 14th, but I was adamant that it could not happen on Valentine's Day. My son was not going to spend the rest of his life catering to girlfriends and his future wife on his big day.

As you would expect, I had the perfect plan for the birth of my first child. I was supposed to check in at the hospital at 11:00 a.m., but I couldn't eat or drink for eight hours before I arrived. So, John and I decided to set the alarm for 2:00 a.m. and have a romantic candlelight breakfast in the dark. After filling our bellies, we would go back to bed and sleep peacefully until 10:00 a.m. I would get up, take a shower, wash my hair, and get my makeup just right for that new mama picture of me holding my newborn son. It was going to be the perfect social media post I'd been waiting for all my life.

Brady, however, had other ideas.

Two days before our appointment, John and I were getting ready to go patio furniture shopping after lunch. I was full of energy that morning. The night before, I had the best night's sleep of my entire life. I remarked to John that, for the first time in months, I was wide awake. I ate a delicious sandwich with some left-over pork tenderloin before we left and had just walked out of our bedroom into our tile-floored entryway when WOOSH! I looked down, and I was soaking wet from the waist down, and there was a small pool of liquid on the floor. My water had broken, which the doctors told us only happens in the movies. And apparently, to me.

We called the doctor, and she said to head to the hospital, so John mobilized quickly. He called my parents to alert them he would be dropping off our beagle and loaded the dog in the car. I went into my room to change out of my soaking wet capri pants. I looked in the mirror and gasped. I hadn't showered in two days! My hair was a greasy mess! I was not photo-ready by any stretch of the imagination! My bag wasn't even fully packed. I stood frozen for a few seconds, deciding what I had time to do before John came back for me. Packing the overnight bag won, hair and makeup lost.

As we pulled into the hospital parking lot we looked for the valet parkers who were supposed to greet us, and then realized it was Sunday. During our tour a couple months earlier, we were told to give the car to the valet parkers, unless it was Sunday. No one was there to take the car, so John told me to go up to the admissions desk on the second floor and he would park and be right behind me.

I grabbed my roller bag, shimmied out of the car, and waddled into the hospital by myself. I pressed the button to call the elevator, and as the doors opened, I walked in with two other visitors. The doors closed and before we could turn around and smile awkwardly at each other, the unthinkable happened—another woosh. My water broke again. Did you know that could happen? I didn't. That was not in my pregnancy books. And it certainly never happened in any movies I'd seen.

I was mortified. The two strangers sharing the four-by-six box looked on in frozen horror. One asked me gently if I was okay and needed help. I whimpered no in response, and when the doors opened, I waddled wide-legged to the admission desk to check-in.

The nurses helped me get undressed, into a gown, and into bed. I instructed them to throw the pants away. I never wanted to see them again. John finally joined me at my bedside, and that's when the contractions started. Contractions were not part of the plan, but I figured they would help me get to the front of the line for the operation room. Instead, I made the mistake of being honest about what I'd eaten that day, and the pork sandwich put me on a nine-hour game delay.

Thankfully Brady made it into the world two and a half hours before becoming the dreaded Valentine baby. John brought Brady over to me and I remember thinking I had never seen eyes so blue in my life. I was strapped to the operating table so I couldn't hold him right away, which didn't seem fair. But John reminded me that due to my incapacitation from the surgery he would be on diaper changing duty for the first 24 hours. That seemed like a good trade.

Brady was born very healthy. He had all ten fingers and toes, working eyes and ears, and no life-threatening conditions, thank the Lord. The first couple of days in the hospital were exhausting and surreal as they are for all new parents.

The first night I couldn't get Brady to stop crying. It was the first of many soul-sucking moments of not feeling qualified to be a mother. The nurse finally came in, grabbed his blanket, and started deftly wrapping it around him like a Chipotle employee wrapping a burrito. She put Brady in the bassinet and he fell right to sleep. I immediately started to cry, "How did you do that??" I blubbered. The nurse smiled sweetly at me and said, "This isn't my first rodeo, sweetie. Now you get some sleep, and I'll show you how to swaddle when you wake up." Looking back, I was grateful God let me have one last good night's sleep. I haven't had one since.

I am still astonished that no one ever told me how hard the first few weeks are at home with a newborn. It must be the best-kept secret in the history of the world. I mean, sure, we know that childbirth itself is no picnic, thanks to Eve's inability to follow the ONE rule God had in the Garden of Eden. But where were our mothers and friends who had kids before us? Why didn't they tell us what really happens when you bring the baby home?

I guess I can understand that my mom didn't want to risk her opportunity to have a grandchild by telling me the truth. I am a second child, and I couldn't understand how anyone could handle two of these creatures, much less more. One particularly hard day, I called my mom in tears and asked her why in the world she decided to have me. She replied flatly, "I didn't want to, but your father insisted." Thanks, Dad.

The world makes us think parenting should look like a Pampers commercial. Everyone is clean and rested. Life is peaceful. The mother is fully confident and equipped to keep this little human alive. In reality, it's a hot mess that is more akin to what fills the Pampers. While I'd expected parenthood to be filled with joy, I didn't expect the full physical, mental, and emotional toll it would take on me.

About a week after Brady was born, John had to go back to work, and I would be alone with Brady for the first time. I hadn't slept for more than thirty minutes in days and wasn't sure how to manage Brady without another pair of eyes and hands. When John walked out of the door to the garage, I was sitting in his recliner chair with the baby on the feeding pillow in my lap, quiet tears slipping down my cheeks. I made it through the day with some help from my mom, but when John finally arrived home about ten hours later, he walked in and saw me in the exact same spot. Poor guy, he made the mistake of commenting, "Wow, you're right where I left you this morning!" As you can imagine, that went poorly for him. I remember sobbing, putting a voice to the thought that kept ripping through my mind, "I thought I would be better at this."

It didn't help that Brady came out of the womb a picky eater, deciding immediately that my breast milk was not cutting it. He wanted to feed every forty-five minutes, and he was not gaining weight like he should. He was too skinny and cranky because he was never full. I was cranky too. Brady was constantly hungry and I was nearly delirious from lack of sleep.

Finally after six weeks, my OB asked me, "Why are you torturing yourself? Give the poor kid a bottle!" It was a difficult decision for me since the world tells us if you don't breastfeed until the kid can walk and talk, you are a failure. But I was desperate. I chalked up another demerit in my internal mommy scorecard and switched to formula. Within days, he plumped right up into a proper Michelin baby, and he and Mama finally got some much-needed rest.

I thought we could get my planning train back on the right track since Brady was no longer "hangry," and I was finally getting some sleep, but we had a few more surprises in store.

When Brady was about two months old, we learned he had severe torticollis, which meant he couldn't turn his head to the right. I felt terrible that we hadn't noticed earlier that he always looked to the left. The treatment involved sessions with an occupational therapist twice a week and daily home exercises four times a day. The home routine was torturous for both of us. I had to grab my new baby's head and twist and hold it to the right for several seconds to stretch the muscle. Of course, he wriggled and cried in pain, and I felt like the worst mom in the world.

Brady also needed to wear a baby helmet for several months to fix the dent in his head, where he leaned up against my rib for several months. The helmet had to be on 23 hours per day, with just an hour off to bathe him. I hated it. I longed to feel the nuzzle of my baby's soft head against my shoulder, but we had to cram all of our snuggling into what my husband termed "the hour of power." We also had to drive to the hospital every week so the helmet could be adjusted. That wouldn't seem like a problem, except Brady HATED being in the car. He screamed bloody murder from the time I put him in the car seat until I took him out. For nearly an hour each way, I was blasted from the back seat with the evidence that I was really not good at this parenting thing.

In between the challenges, we had moments of great joy and gratitude with Brady. But deep down, I felt cheated. My perfect plan to be the perfect mother and to have the perfect parenting experience had been blown to smithereens, and I was only a few months in.

What I had not learned yet is there is no such thing as a perfect plan. In fact, it's an oxymoron like jumbo shrimp. The only way a plan can come to fruition perfectly is if you are in control of all the variables, which I was not. None of us are. The only one in the universe whose plans can work is God because He is the only one who has real control. The Bible even tells us that man plans, but the LORD's purpose will prevail (Proverbs 19:21). So if a perfect human plan does come together, it is only because God lets it be so.

My resentment for my situation also highlighted that I had an entitlement problem. I felt like I deserved the Pampers commercial because I planned for it. I felt robbed because I had a false sense of ownership of a future that was not mine yet. It was okay for me to have a vision of what I wanted for my future, but when my joy was dependent on adherence to my plan, I was destined for disappointment. I needed a more solid, foundational basis for joy that couldn't be shaken when my plans fell apart.

I was about to learn that the hard way.

CHAPTER 2
FROM DRiZZLE TO DOWNPOUR

My first brush with autism occurred when I was about six months pregnant with Brady. It's almost hard to fathom now that autism is such a huge part of my life. But at the time, I knew nothing about the diagnosis, and only related autism to Dustin Hoffman's character in the movie *Rainman*.

I was participating in a women's networking group, and a new member asked me to lunch to discuss our businesses. She was a pretty blonde, a little younger than I, but when we settled at our table I could tell she was shy and not sure how to get the conversation started. I asked about her family, figuring it was an easy topic to get her to open up.

Alison told me she was a single mom with two boys, one of whom had autism. I was curious, so I asked her what her son was like. She told me Alex was eleven and could name every major league baseball player, his team, position, and batting average. I thought that was amazing—what a memory he must have! But then she went on to tell me about his struggles at school and home. Alex had severe anxiety and would have outbursts in the classroom on a regular basis, so she was constantly getting called away from work to deal with it. He was being bullied by other children and was having a really hard time keeping up academically, even though she knew he was very smart. Alex had no friends, but she was thankful he had a little brother so he wasn't completely alone.

I could see the pain on her face as she talked about her son's challenges. She obviously needed help, and someone to talk to considering she was pouring her heart out to a total stranger.

I wanted to comfort her, but I didn't know how. I just listened, acknowledging her situation was difficult, but offering no advice or counsel. I was not that person, I thought. Not yet.

After that lunch, autism became my biggest fear in pregnancy. It was a persistent, annoying thought that kept creeping into my psyche even through Brady's toddlerhood. I was relieved at Brady's two-year well-check exam when we got the "all clear" from his pediatrician. "No autism," she told us. He walked on time at one, talked on time at two, so I could finally put that irrational notion behind me.

Ironically, it was around the time when autism was supposedly off the table when other things about Brady's behavior started setting a new table of concern.

For instance, at our "mommy-and-me" classes, everyone was supposed to sit in a circle with her child on her lap while we sang the welcome ditty. Brady would have nothing to do with the circle, so I would have to follow him around the gymnastics equipment until the song was over. If the class was on the balance beam, Brady was trying to figure out how to connect the hose for the bouncy pad to the air pump. One of the moms politely pointed out that Brady was probably going to be an engineer someday because he was more interested in the mechanics of how the machine worked than bouncing on it.

Playdates were another source of frustration for me. I met a nice group of moms in the neighborhood, and we often gathered with the children; only Brady had no interest in playing with their kids. If we were at someone's home, Brady would go to the door and try to leave. If we were at a playground or park, he would position himself on the furthest perimeter to maximize the distance between him and the group of kids we were there to see. He needed constant supervision, while the other kids could just play together endlessly.

The worst part? I was missing out on all the conversations with the other moms while I chased Brady, trying unsuccessfully to convince him to join the group. I used to joke that I should get a babysitter for playdates, although it wasn't really a joke.

The other moms were kind, but I could see friendships blooming in the garden of their conversations while I was stuck on the other side of the fence. I had planned to make lifelong friends through this stage of Brady's life, but it wasn't going to happen when I only caught bits and pieces of discussions as I ran by in hot pursuit of my son. Even though they gave me no reason to, I imagined the other ladies talking about Brady and me. Wondering why Brady wouldn't play with their kids, and wondering what I was doing wrong as a parent for him to act this way.

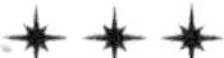

When Brady started preschool at age two, his developmental differences started to become more pronounced as we were able to compare him to other children on a daily basis. He cried every day at drop off, without fail. While other kids were making friends, he couldn't even tell us the names of his classmates. His teachers would send pictures at the end of the day, and when the class was in a circle, Brady was on his back in the corner of the room with his legs in the air, in what John affectionately called "the cockroach."

At home, there were some behaviors emerging that, in hindsight, I should have realized were not typical. Brady was completely obsessed with *The Wiggles.* For those of you who have not had the pleasure of seeing an episode of *The Wiggles,* it was four grown Australian men who would sing, dance, and cavort with Dorothy the Dinosaur, Wags the Dog, and Captain Feathersword, the friendly pirate. But it wasn't just the episodes that interested Brady; it was the DVD covers.

Each DVD cover had a paper inset with pictures of *The Wiggles* on it, and on the back cover, they advertised other *Wiggles* DVDs with small miniature pictures of those DVD covers. Brady would lay each box on the ottoman and look at them intently, rocking back and forth, sometimes not even watching the show playing on TV. Eventually, just looking at the covers wasn't enough for him – he wanted to get to the paper under the clear cover. My organized brain didn't want the insets to get wrinkled and torn in his little fingers, so I had a great idea: I copied the cover page, put the original back in the plastic cover, and then taped it shut. Brilliant.

But Brady decided there was a lot on the black and white page that didn't interest him, so he asked us to cut out certain pieces of the copy. Sometimes it was Jeff's head, or Murray's guitar, or one of the mini-DVD advertisements on the back. He would hold these little pieces of paper like they were gold. If he lost one, it was a tragedy until the paper could get pulled out again, copied, cut, and life could get back to normal.

There were lots of other hints that should have prompted us to dig deeper. He could not ride a bike or catch a ball to save his life. *So, he won't be an athlete,* I thought. *Big deal. He'll probably be a math whiz.* He wouldn't snuggle with me when I would read him a story, and in fact, he almost always needed something else to do during story time. *He's just a multitasker like his mom,* I mused. He buried himself between the back of our couch and the heavy down cushions on a regular basis and sometimes refused to come out. *Okay, we just need to get him a comfier bed.* The Vitamix blender would send him into a screaming panic. *Yes, it was loud; maybe all kids have more sensitive hearing than adults?* We rationalized everything that should have been a warning sign.

These observations were swirling around in my head with no real direction. I was concerned, but I didn't know if I was overreacting. *After all, every kid develops at a different pace, right?*

For John and me, it was like we were getting sprinkled with gentle rain, unaware that a downpour was ready to start.

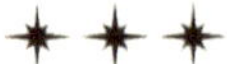

One summer day, when Brady was three, John and I took Brady to an indoor trampoline park with my best friend's family. I was watching Brady and their daughter who was the same age, as they jumped in a dodgeball court that was enclosed with plexiglass. As usual, Brady was in his own world on the far edge of the room, but suddenly, a boy about nine or ten years old grabbed my friend's little girl by her head and started pounding it into the clear plastic. For a split second I froze, not believing what my eyes were seeing. Then I snapped into action as instinct took over my body. I immediately ran to her and roughly pulled the boy away from her. I pushed him behind me as I picked her up and she started to cry.

She wasn't really hurt, but shocked and scared, as was I. Holding her in one hand, I extended my arm toward the boy, telling him in no uncertain terms to stay away.

Out of the corner of my eye, I saw a man running toward the court, yelling, "Curtis! Curtis!" When he got closer, I heard him say, "I'm so sorry, is she okay? He doesn't know what he's doing. He has Aspergers." I didn't know what Aspergers was at the time, and I didn't care. It sounded like an excuse for bad parenting, and I was not the picture of grace at that moment. No, I was the picture of judgment, shame, and anger. Instead of putting myself in that father's shoes and understanding that he was doing the best he could with a child who didn't know how to regulate emotions, I retorted, "Well then, maybe you shouldn't leave him alone with other kids." Ouch, I know. To make that family's humiliation complete, John went to tell the manager the family needed to be kicked out of the facility.

God, forgive us. If only we knew what life would be like for our family just a few weeks later when Brady would be diagnosed with the Exact. Same. Thing. How's that for irony? Turns out Aspergers is a form of autism, and while it is not specifically diagnosed using the Aspergers terminology anymore, it is part of the "spectrum" with which we would become so intimately familiar.

I like to think that one-month-older me would have responded differently, with more compassion and grace. My reaction belittled that boy and his father. It elevated me to some imaginary high horse without the slightest regard for their feelings. That was a tough lesson to learn and one that I would revisit each time I found myself in Curtis's dad's position. And believe me, I have been there. Thankfully, Brady has never physically hurt anyone else, but I have felt the weight of the stares and comments of strangers who were unaware of our family's situation.

One good thing came out of the experience—I call it the Three-Hour Rule. Maybe it can help you too. The next time you see a mother or father who is hanging by a thread, please don't snip it loose with a misplaced air of superiority. Remember, you are witnessing a single, culminating moment. You have no perspective or context to make sense of the situation. Instead, consider what the last three hours might have been like. If she is at the end of her rope now, she has probably been sliding down steadily for some time. As the parent of an autistic child who has had to manage her son in the throes of a tantrum in front of strangers, I wished other people could understand what had transpired before they entered the scene.

Whether it was three hours ago, three minutes ago, or three years ago, every person you meet is carrying something that you can't see, and it is impacting how they interact with you. Your cashier at the grocery store, the person driving next to you, the waiter at the restaurant, if you can't see Jesus in them, they might need to see Jesus in you. Understand that three hours ago might have rocked their world, and you are seeing the rubble.

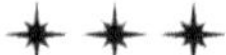

It was in the weeks after the incident with Curtis that all the sprinkles of concern started to turn into a storm.

One morning after another meltdown at preschool dropoff, I decided to ask his teacher if she had any concerns. She had no problem coming up with several, including the circle time avoidance, lack of relational skills with his peers, and inability to answer direct questions. She didn't have any recommendations for me, other than assurances he would be fine. I wasn't so sure.

My "mommy radar" was starting to beep. Loudly. I was distracted on the drive home, trying to figure out what I should do next. When I got home, I sat down in my office to work, but I had a hard time concentrating. I absentmindedly picked up a magazine from my desk and started to look through it. It was a free local edition that I usually tossed in recycling without even opening the cover. The pages were full of fashion articles and pictures of the town's elite at charity fundraisers, so I never paid much attention. To this day, I believe God put that magazine in my hands to open my eyes.

As I flipped carelessly through the ads and photos, I found an article called "A Mission to Help." It told the story of Patty Dion, whose son Dave was diagnosed with Asperger's Disorder, but not until he was an adult. As I read the article, my stomach began to turn. Patty's description of her son at Brady's age was frighteningly familiar: little interaction with peers, trouble performing various life tasks, poor social skills, difficulty understanding social cues, odd or limited interests, and problems making friends.

At the end of the article, there was a link to an online quiz to see if your child had enough characteristics to warrant a professional evaluation. I didn't pause—I went directly to the link. The DAVE questionnaire (Detecting Asperger's Very Early) was developed by the Southwest Autism Research & Resource Center (SARRC) and was a list of fifteen simple yes or no questions. The pit in my stomach started to grow exponentially as I answered "Yes" over and over again. By the time I clicked "Submit," there was no question in my mind what the answer would be.

"The results of the DAVE Screening Questionnaire indicate the need for a formal assessment for Autism Spectrum Disorder."

There it was. We didn't have a diagnosis yet, but I was certain. The drizzle of awareness had opened up into a full thunderstorm that would threaten the stability of the very ground on which I stood.

CHAPTER 3
PLATE SHiFTiNG

In January 1994, I found myself on unsteady ground for a different reason. I had recently graduated from college and was living my dream life in Hermosa Beach, California. I worked for an investment advisory firm in Los Angeles, and the window of my cubicle looked out at the Hollywood sign. I spent my weekend days at the beach, and at night my financially challenged friends and I would track down the best happy hour deals which provided the most amount of free food for the least amount of money.

I had lived in California for about six months when I experienced my first earthquake. I was at a friend's house when we felt her apartment start shifting, very gently, side to side. It reminded me of being in a car and letting the tires roll up and down on a speed bump. The movement only lasted a few seconds before stillness resumed, and I wasn't the least bit rattled. In fact, I thought it was cool! I considered this minor quake my initiation into California living.

It turns out that was just the preamble. About a week later, I woke up early one morning, not sure what stirred me from sleep. Then, the shaking started. This was not a little shimmy. It felt like a giant had picked up the entire apartment complex and started shaking it violently like a kid who was trying to determine the contents of a Christmas present. I sat up on my elbow, unsure of what to do, when my roommate threw open my bedroom door and screamed at me to get into the doorframe. But I didn't move. In my failed logic, I thought I would be safer lying in bed because if the floors above me collapsed, I would just get squished into my soft mattress and be okay. By the way, that is NOT the recommended procedure in case you ever find yourself in a similar situation.

The violent pounding continued for so long that I could not fathom how the building hadn't yet crumbled around us. The large, heavy mirror attached to the wall over my dresser crashed to the ground. My clothes in the closet looked like they were going through an agitation cycle in a washer. I could hear clanging as appliances jumped on the kitchen counter. Finally, the trembling tapered off, and we were left with the sound of car alarms and sirens piercing the early morning. I got up slowly and surveyed the apartment. It was a wreck, but thankfully, all four walls and ceiling were still intact.

As the adrenaline rush started to wane, fear set in. Then my phone rang.

My dad had an early morning meeting that day and woke up to the real-time news of the massive earthquake. When I heard his voice, I started to cry. I was terrified the shaking would start again. I pictured getting sucked into a crack in the ground and falling to my death in the earth's core. Dad tried to calm me down and encouraged me to get dressed and go to work. After all, he reminded me, I was the low man on the totem pole in a new job, and it was important to show my bosses my commitment to the organization. In his defense, he had no idea how destructive the quake had been. There were no reports of damage yet, and he was trying to get my focus off the terror of the last few minutes and back to normalcy.

I hung up with him and sniffled softly as I went to shower so I could get ready for work like a good soldier. But when I reached for the faucet, the water wouldn't turn on. *I guess I'll have to rely on deodorant,* I thought. I got dressed and walked to my car with the sound of different alarms still blaring relentlessly in a dissonant chorus. As I pulled out of my complex onto Pacific Coast Highway, the reality of the aftermath started to set in. Streetlights were out. The glass showrooms of the car dealerships were blown out, and I started to notice that I was the only one on the road. Finally, survival instinct took over my desire to show my corporate responsibility, and I turned around and drove home. Turns out it was the right move. My route to work passed directly under the stretch of Interstate 10 which had buckled and collapsed.

My office building was closed until structural engineers could inspect it, so we got a few extra days off until they deemed it safe for us to return. There were several significant aftershocks in the days that followed. It was bad enough to feel the shaking at home, but I worked on the 22nd floor of a high rise. When they reopened the office after almost a week, I was scared to death to be up that high when the earth was not secure beneath me. California natives tried to calm my nerves by explaining the buildings sat on rollers, but just like my roommate's instruction to get in the doorway, this architectural earthquake logic escaped me.

As if to test my disbelief, the first day back at work we had a huge aftershock, and the whole building started to sway like those inflatable figures that draw attention to used car lots. It was nauseating. Job or no job, I couldn't take it anymore. Fight or flight took over, and flight won. I ran to the door, rode down the elevator, jumped into my car, and after a quick stop to pick up some clothes, I set my course for a nice, steady Arizona.

If you had asked me on the seven-hour car ride if I would ever return to the land of shake, rattle, and roll, I would have answered a resounding "no." But a few days of shake-free downtime with Mom and Dad calmed my nerves, and I missed the beach. My boss had been very understanding, but it was time to put on my big girl pants and go back to work. I did so knowing that what I once thought was an immutable law of the universe—secure ground—was now a privilege, not a guarantee.

After realizing that all signs pointed to Brady having autism, my world started to shake again, but this time, the quake was in my soul. I was shell-shocked. I was unsure of my footing, not trusting the very ground I was standing on.

I think my mom, using her ESP superpower, must have sensed I was in danger because she called me just minutes after I took the fateful quiz. It may surprise you to know I live three blocks away from my parents. Before you judge me for making my poor husband live so close to his in-laws, I'll have you know it was his idea. When we found the house, I was pregnant with Brady, and John very rightly assumed that having grandparents/babysitters so close to us would be helpful. That was the understatement of the century.

When my mom heard my voice, she could tell something was wrong, and I think it was about 90 seconds from the time I choked out my suspicions until my Dad was at my door.

We didn't make it out of the entryway before I collapsed in his arms, crying from the deepest place in my gut. He continued to hold me up and squeeze me tightly, but this time, not even the safety of my Dad's embrace could make things stable again. All I could think about was Curtis, the boy in the trampoline park. Would Brady end up like him? Then, other doubts started flowing in like a waterfall. Could he go to school? Would he be able to have a job? Move out? Get married?

In a matter of minutes all the dreams I had for Brady's future became as unstable as the ground in an earthquake. This was so much more than a failed plan. It felt like God picked up the box of my life and shook it so hard I couldn't recognize it anymore.

I don't know how long Dad and I stood there, but eventually, I pulled away and tried to wipe away the tears that hadn't already soaked Dad's shirt. We said our goodbyes, but not without Dad promising he and my mom would help however they could. I knew he meant it.

Alone once again, I realized I only had a little time before I had to pick Brady up at school. I had to resume normal mommy duties for the next seven hours until he went to bed and I could talk to John about my discoveries.

John. When I kissed him goodbye this morning, we were just parents with nagging worries. Over the next few hours, the earth made a tectonic shift under my feet, but John was still on a firm foundation.

I wasn't sure how John would take it. I thought there was a chance he would reject the idea that Brady had autism, say I was reading too much into it, say we just needed to give him time to grow out of it, or any other number of excuses to deny the truth of which I had become so certain.

It was one of those "we need to talk" moments everyone dreads in life. After Brady went to sleep, I settled into the couch, and John reclined in his chair and listened quietly as I recounted the events of the day. As I explained the questionnaire, the discussion with his teacher, and the small amount of research I had time to find before picking Brady up, I was like a lawyer delivering closing arguments. It all culminated in my conclusion: Brady has autism. John looked at me and didn't object, and he didn't fight. He just took it all in and responded, "OK. So what do we do now?"

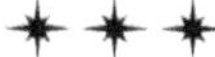

John and I committed to each other we would do whatever it took to help Brady have the best chance at a fulfilling and productive life. Brady was priority one, and speed was of the essence. He would be four in a few months, and some studies we read concluded that after he turned five the efficacy of treatment would fall dramatically. The pressure was immense, and we encountered numerous wait lists when we tried to schedule appointments for intervention. When we finally got the formal medical diagnosis a couple of months later, we had already piecemealed a combination of various therapies.

We focused all our energy on trying to find the right blend that would have the most positive impact on his future. But autism is so different for each child that there was no formula I could follow. I didn't have a roadmap that showed how to get from where we were to where we wanted to be. We were throwing lots of spaghetti at the wall, hoping some strands would stick.

The internet websites for parents of newly diagnosed children recommended speech, occupational, and physical therapy, as well as twenty to forty hours per week of Applied Behavioral Analysis, or ABA therapy. Brady's preschool gave us access to a speech therapist right away, and the OT who helped us when he was a baby, for the torticollis, squeezed us into weekly sessions. It felt good that we were doing something, but it didn't feel like nearly enough. And the clock was ticking.

Filling out intake forms became a full-time job. Each agency had thick stacks of documents that needed to be printed and completed by hand with the same information over and over again. Details about my pregnancy and Brady's birth, dates of Brady's firsts—rolling over, walking, talking, and sentences. Surveys about his behaviors, interests, sensory needs, and social interaction. Each one highlighted some seemingly innocuous trait that is apparently a giant red flag for autism.

John is a spreadsheet ninja, so he started keeping data of all the therapies Brady completed in a week. After we hit the thousand-hour mark, we stopped keeping track. Thankfully, most of the therapy sessions were play-based, and Brady enjoyed the focused attention from adults, especially the little rewards he could earn, like stickers, candy, and small plastic toys that slowly started to overtake our home. He never asked me why he had to go to so many appointments. He didn't know any better. But I did.

I saw my friends with kids Brady's age who were living Facebook-fabulous lives filled with activities and milestones I was missing. I knew I should be grateful for all the things my son could do, but I think deep down, I believed if we worked hard enough, we could put this whole autism thing behind us before he went to kindergarten. The further we got from the diagnosis, the further the imaginary finish line slipped away until it completely disappeared. I wanted a finish line. I needed a finish line.

I put on a good show for outsiders, but I became disengaged and irritable with those closest to me. I felt like a hamster in a wheel, running constantly in circles with no final destination in sight. My world got rocked with an online quiz, and my perfect plan tumbled into the abyss.

When an earthquake occurs, the tectonic plates shift far beneath the surface, and they never go back to where they started. They settle into their new location until the next shift comes. The same thing happens when your life gets shaken. You never land in the same place either. You can spend a lot of time and energy trying to get back to where you were, but the pieces won't fit. The plans you made before aren't possible or won't make sense from your new position.

Most of the challenges we face don't have clear-cut solutions, like a victory, a cure, or a reversal of fortune that can bring you back to the starting line. When the shaking stops, our plate will be on new ground. We need to find something so strong and steady that no matter what happens to the ground beneath us, we have something to hold on to. Without it, we will be stuck riding the shockwaves.

I was tired of riding the waves. I needed to find some solid rock, but I wasn't sure where to look.

CHAPTER 4
SHAME iS A SUCKER

For the first few years after the diagnosis, John and I were swimming in the deep end of autism, but we did our best to make sure it was a private pool. Only our family, a few close friends, and his preschool teachers knew of Brady's actual diagnosis for the first few years. We made a pact that we would not speak the word autism in the house, around Brady, or in front of anyone who was not part of our circle of trust. If someone asked what was going on with Brady, we would say he had some "developmental delays." Even if I was speaking to a medical provider or close family, I never said Brady had autism or that he was autistic. I said he was "diagnosed" with autism. The difference may seem subtle, but saying he had autism was acknowledgment and acceptance of his condition. Just being diagnosed didn't mean it was real.

Why the secrecy? Fear was a factor. We were afraid of so many things. We were concerned that other parents with the same limited knowledge we had about autism would want to keep their kids away from Brady. Our interaction with Curtis at the trampoline park was fresh in our minds. I hate to admit it, but if Curtis had been my only exposure to autism, I would probably want to keep Brady away from other autistic children, too.

We also worried he would be permanently "labeled" and would be kept from future opportunities or careers. John is a West Point graduate, and he assumed Brady might be excluded from military service with autism on his medical record. We didn't even tell the school district at first, unsure if he would end up ostracized and isolated from other kids.

We thought we could keep Brady's autism to ourselves until he eventually grew out of it. We clung to that hope as we raced from therapy to therapy, unwilling to admit autism was more than a temporary condition.

It wasn't just fear, though, at least for me. Fear was a big part, but there was a twinge of shame that kept me from admitting I had a son with special needs. I wasn't ashamed of Brady, not in the slightest. I was ashamed of myself. I was ashamed I had failed to produce a human who was a perfect fit for the world around me. I was ashamed I hadn't recognized his autism earlier. I was ashamed I couldn't participate in the same motherhood club as my friends with neurotypical children.

Shame is a sucker, feeding on its host and slowly extracting the person we were, replacing us with an actor following a script. To keep up appearances, we put on a happy face, downplay our weaknesses, and hide. If you are like me, you want people to think the very best of you, but shame makes you feel like a poser. You feel exposed, just waiting for someone to pull back the curtain. That's why some of us rely so heavily on our own plans. If we can control all the variables, if we can make our plan work, we won't be revealed as who we really are. Sometimes, the instinct to want to plan is just a symptom of a greater problem—the need to be an achiever, a winner, and an example to others.

When it came to motherhood, I wanted to be all three. But in my mind, I was none of the above.

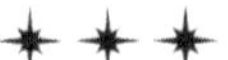

Our initial decision not to involve the school district was a rookie mistake, and the psychologist who diagnosed Brady encouraged us to get an educational assessment right away. If it was determined that Brady's autism would impact his experience in the classroom, we could take advantage of some federally mandated services and resources. In addition, Arizona has a robust school-choice platform, and based on the district evaluation, if the public school was not right for him, we could be eligible to receive funds to attend private schools.

It took a couple of months to get the "Comprehensive Developmental Assessment" scheduled. John had to work, so I brought Brady at the appointed time to an elementary school gym, where several tiny makeshift rooms were partitioned with sheets hanging on wheeled racks. I had completed the lengthy intake forms and parent surveys in advance, and they had also visited Brady's preschool to observe him in the classroom. I waited nervously on a plastic folding chair as different teachers guided Brady through the sections for testing.

After about an hour, the assessment culminated in a round table discussion with six education professionals I'd never met. Each took turns rattling off test scores that may as well have been in another language. They tested Brady for Cognitive, Social-Emotional, Adaptive, Speech & Language, and Physical Development, including fine and gross motor skills. While they spoke, Brady was crawling under the table, pulling at my legs. I tried to take notes, but I didn't understand the lingo, and I was trying to manage Brady, so all I captured was a recurring theme—delayed. Before the last educator could complete his report, Brady started screaming like someone had stuck knives in his belly. He was done. I picked him up and held him in my lap, rocking back and forth furiously, missing everything the speaker said. I felt the entire gym staring at us as tears welled in my eyes.

Someone finally told us we could go. I grabbed Brady and my purse, and before we walked out, a woman pulled me aside and reiterated the summary of the assessment: Brady was developmentally delayed. With an autism diagnosis, that was not a surprise, but now the school system had identified how those delays would impact his ability to learn in a traditional educational environment.

The good news? We were eligible for services. Lots of them. We would have to wait another month before the final report was ready, but the team told me Brady could start attending the developmental preschool at one of the local elementary schools, known as "PANDA." PANDA stands for the "Program for Assessed Needs in All Developmental Areas." It was a half-day school, four days per week, and there was no cost for him to attend. In addition, he would receive small amounts of speech therapy, occupational therapy, and physical therapy each week, also at no charge. Private therapy could be very expensive, so these programs are essential to some families.

A woman invited me to take a tour of the PANDA classroom and said Brady could start as soon as the Individualized Education Plan (IEP) was completed and agreed upon by all parties. It sounded perfect. Free services, and we could keep Brady in his original preschool in the morning, send him to PANDA in the afternoon, and continue additional therapies after school. For some reason, it gave me comfort that more of Brady's day would be consumed with activity. It felt productive.

John came with me for the tour. We arrived at the school and were greeted warmly by the assistant principal, who showed us to the classroom. When we went inside, I felt a knot form in my stomach. There were about seven or eight other children, all boys, most of them severely impacted. One child was in a stroller and was grunting, seemingly unaware of the activity around him. Others were yelling out or exhibiting behaviors that were aggressive and disconcerting. The teacher had to use a microphone to communicate. It was a very different scene than the one I was used to at Brady's preschool.

As my breath quickened, I had the sudden urge to run from the room. Was this my son's future? Did he belong there? I knew that he needed the assistance that the school district was willing to provide, but it was not the expectation I had for his preschool experience. For the first but not the last time, I was using my pre-autism vision of what Brady's life was supposed to be to shape my decision-making process. What I wanted and what Brady needed were rarely going to be the same thing.

On the way to the car, I shared my apprehension with John. He saw it differently. He was impressed with the teacher and the mechanisms they had in place to work with the children and felt none of the foreboding that had flooded into my psyche. He reminded me that Brady needed help, and they were professionals with the capacity to provide it. John thought we needed to give PANDA a try, and I reluctantly agreed.

About two months after starting the new preschool, Brady started coming home with even more dramatic behaviors. He started to bang his head against the wall or the counter when he got frustrated. He was moaning and pulling at the tuft of hair above his forehead. We feared he was regressing, even though the teacher's reports were positive. And the services he was allotted according to the IEP were minimal—some only 30 minutes per week.

As the school semester ended, we decided that it was time to move on. We were grateful that the district provided the school for kids with conditions that required more assistance, but Brady fell somewhere in between. He needed more support than a mainstream classroom would give him but didn't fit into the self-contained classroom model either. He was in the gap. It was time to boil some more spaghetti and let it fly.

The next couple of years were a blur of evaluations, therapies, parent training, and in-home treatment. We were instructed by his developmental pediatrician to keep Brady around neurotypical children as much as possible so they could model expected behavior for him. We loved his preschool, but it was becoming more and more difficult for him to get through the day with his peers without significant intervention from his teachers.

The preschool agreed to let us have an aide in Brady's classroom, and we found a delightful woman with a heart for special kids who became his buddy. Julie was a true Godsend. She loved Brady and was adept at making his classmates think she was there to help them all. She kept Brady on task, helped him in social situations with the other kids, and facilitated breaks when he needed them. She used his intense interests to create powerful teaching aides that helped Brady learn things that came naturally to other kids.

At home, we made a startling realization that Brady was unable to interpret others' feelings. One night, our beagle Bailey, who had multiple health issues, was having an episode we thought would force us to put him down. As we waited for my parents to come by to watch Brady so we could take Bailey to the vet, I was sitting on the kitchen floor, holding the dog in my lap and crying. Brady just kept coming up to me with his *Wiggles* DVD cover, saying, "Copy Mommy, copy Mommy." I replied, "Brady, Mommy is really sad because Bailey is very sick. I can't make a copy right now." Brady just got more adamant, "Copy, Mommy, copy!" He was oblivious. I remember sitting on that cold tile crying, and it dawned on me that either he didn't recognize that I was in pain or he didn't care. I prayed it was the former.

Most of Brady's negative behaviors were almost exclusively directed at me. We spent a lot of time alone together, and I was his safe person. When he became dysregulated, his three-year-old brain would come up with wild, destructive scenarios of how I would be removed from his life. I should have known then that creative writing would be one of his gifts because the stories were always very detailed and elaborate. We realized much later that those outbursts were self-punishing behaviors—not directed at me. He was preparing himself to lose me somehow, but knowledge of the purpose of his words didn't make them sting any less.

Thankfully, he never lashed out at another child or family member, but that made it difficult for John and my family to understand the severity of his condition. I learned to take notes after episodes so I could explain to John what had happened while he was at work. If I didn't write it down immediately afterward, it would just be a foggy account summed up as: "We had a bad day."

On the bright side, during this time we also observed Brady's true personality emerge. He loved dancing to *The Wiggles* and would bounce fervently on our couch, copying the hand gestures of his Australian friends. When he got excited about something, he would jump up and down, flapping his wrists so hard I sometimes thought they would disconnect from his arm. He loved being with family, and we noted that with us, the people closest to him, he could look us right in the eye.

We also discovered Brady's love of performing. He had no fear of a microphone or large crowds. It was surprising considering his autism, but perfectly natural considering his mom. I didn't get the nickname Karaoke Kari for nothing.

At his kindergarten talent show, he played "Ode to Joy" by Beethoven with one hand on an electric keyboard in front of a large crowd of over 100 parents. He walked onstage with the confidence that can only come from someone with no concern for others' opinions. When he finished the song, the crowd erupted in applause. Only Brady wasn't done. He got up, walked over to the emcee, snatched the microphone out of his hands, and announced his second song, one he wrote called "Chicken Noodle Soup." I'm not sure where the song title came from since he'd never even tried chicken noodle soup. But again, he wowed the crowd, and it was obvious he was in his element.

All along, John and I kept our secret close. There were times we could fake it and get by. I remember the relief I would feel after a gathering with no meltdown or escape attempt. Other times, we felt like Brady's autism was on full display for the world to see and were sure we would be called out.

Shame kept chipping away. When shame replaces your persona with a false front for the rest of the world, it leaves a vacuum when the actor leaves the stage. The hole shame leaves in your soul longs to be filled with something. Lots of people fill it with food, alcohol, or mind-numbing television. I tried it all, but nothing worked. The shame was my problem, not Brady's. I didn't know it at the time, but I was having a crisis of identity that could only be solved by the One who made me.

CHAPTER 5
EQUiP-MENT

Immediately after John and I got engaged, John started researching dog breeds to find the perfect pooch to start our family. We loved looking at puppy pictures online, but even though the sad eyes tugged at our heartstrings from the monitor, we agreed to wait to take the plunge into dog ownership until we'd enjoyed our carefree newlywed life for a few months.

When I say "we" agreed to wait, I may have misstated. Three weeks after our honeymoon, my phone rang while I was on a business trip in Reno. I was meeting with some colleagues from my company, and when I saw it was John, I excused myself to see what was up. It was unusual for him to call me in the middle of a workday.

We said hello, and I could tell he was driving, "Guess what I have on my lap?" John asked. I knew my husband well enough to know it was an innocent question. I decided to cut right to the chase, "What?" You guessed it, it was a dog.

In my absence, John had been spending his free time scouring the internet for a puppy who needed a forever home, and he found one on Craigslist he couldn't resist. Bailey was a three-year-old beagle who had been abandoned and relocated from a shelter in Las Vegas. The foster family taking care of Bailey had a pit bull mama with nine new puppies, so they needed to find a home for Bailey ASAP.

"He was free!" John exclaimed, "They even gave me a leash." *Hmmm, is free a good thing? What happened to getting what you pay for?*

"I'm on my way to the pet store to get some food. Also, the lady said if it doesn't work out, we can bring him back, so it's like a risk-free trial." *Right*, I thought. *I'm sure he threw that last bit in to counter my expected resistance.* I will admit I was a little excited, and it was heartwarming that my new husband was so interested in starting our family. But I was also nervous. John and I hadn't had pets since we were kids. Plus, I was disappointed that our footloose and fancy-free honeymoon period was over so soon.

When I walked through the door at about 10 that night, our new dog ran up to greet me joyfully, and I couldn't help but fall in love with him instantly. Bailey was a lemon beagle, so his fur was only tan and white, not black. His ears were floppy, and his hound dog eyes were filled with emotion. Mostly I noticed that Bailey was extremely overweight. His torso looked like an overstuffed sausage, and his skinny little legs didn't look strong enough to hold his girth. Apparently the foster family had a tub of food out back, and Bailey had a hard time walking away when he was full. Boy, could I relate. We were made for each other.

We played on the floor with him and reveled in our new parent roles. Bailey was overjoyed and wagged his tail so hard I thought it would fly off like a helicopter. He tried to kiss us repeatedly, but we resisted, conscious of where that tongue had been. John called me "Mommy" in front of Bailey, and it melted my heart. Bailey was our first baby.

When it was time to turn in, we didn't have a dog bed for Bailey. We put down some towels on the carpet in our room and tried to encourage him to lie down, but he wouldn't settle in. The happy, tail-wagging bundle of joy I met earlier that night transformed into a trembling, terrified, whining bundle of nerves. I tried to comfort him and snuggled with him on the floor, but nothing worked, and no one slept. It was more like having a baby than we bargained for.

The next morning John left for work early, and although I was bleary-eyed and groggy, I was excited to take Bailey for his first official walk. I couldn't wait to introduce our neighbors to our newest family member, but it would have to wait as the streets were empty. When we got back it was time for me to leave for work.

John and I decided to keep Bailey in the laundry room behind a gate while we were gone. We put more towels on the floor and filled a water bowl, and hoped his exhaustion from the all-nighter would cause him to curl up for a long nap. I coaxed him inside with a tasty treat, but when I closed the gate, he immediately voiced his displeasure. He was yelping a constant high-pitched cry at a decibel level that threatened to pierce my ear drum. I spoke soothingly to him, petted him, but every time I walked out the door his panicked shrieks intensified.

By now, I was in danger of being late for work, and I had to leave. I prayed he would calm down or wear himself out, but even after I put the garage door down, I could still hear him.

Work was a futile effort. I was exhausted and couldn't concentrate, so at lunch I came home and walked into a doggie crime scene.

The gate to the laundry room was down, and the door looked like it had been shredded by Freddy Kruger. I walked into the living room, and there was dog poo everywhere. I couldn't even imagine where it came from—the dog only had one meal since we got him, but it looked like he'd been storing up for weeks. I decided the priority was to make sure we didn't add to the mess, so I grabbed the leash and took him out for a walk.

That's when I learned that besides severe separation anxiety, Bailey suffered from his own social disorder—he hated other dogs. As we passed another unsuspecting neighbor with a dog, Bailey quickly morphed into a forty-pound version of Cujo. He lurched at the unsuspecting dog, barking and pulling at his leash so hard that I dropped the poo bags. He pulled relentlessly on the collar around his neck and I was afraid I was going to choke him to death, so I awkwardly picked up the wriggling monster and carried him home. I found a piece of carpet without poo on it and collapsed in a heap of sweat and tears.

Clearly I was not cut out to be a fur mama! Dogs are supposed to bring their owners joy, not suffering! Plus, if I can't handle a dog, how am I supposed to handle a child?? I spiraled into a pit of self-doubt that was only exacerbated by the smell in the room that I knew wouldn't go away until I got up and started cleaning. I never went back to work that day and wondered if I would have to quit and be a stay-at-home dog mom.

When John walked in I pummeled him with the details of the day from doggy hell. He saw how distraught I was and asked if I wanted to give the dog back to the foster family. That startled me. I hadn't even thought of that. Of course not, I told him. I was already in love with that dysfunctional dog, so there was no way I could give him up. But I was dreading the next ten years of poop and puppy aggression he was going to put us through. No, Bailey was part of our family. We just had to figure out how to parent him better. And we did. Eventually Bailey learned to sleep in a crate and walk on a leash, and while he still preferred humans to other dogs, he was an irreplaceable part of our family.

Dog ownership turned out to be a foreshadowing of my parenting experience. The tantrums, the sad moments, the obsessive interests, and the social delays were foreign to me. I had no clue how to respond or how to help Brady. I felt grossly ill-equipped to be the mom of a kid with special needs. Don't get me wrong, Brady was the source of the best and most complete joy in my life, but on so many occasions, I questioned whether God made a mistake placing Brady in my care.

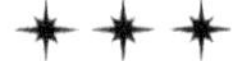

When John and I learned that Brady had autism, it added a level of complexity to parenting that seemed overwhelming. All of a sudden, the stakes seemed higher than ever. Our missteps were not just funny stories that we would tell around the table at Thanksgiving when Brady was grown up. We felt the weight of the world on our shoulders. If we didn't get him the right therapies at the right time, it would have an exponential impact on his probability of success later in life. And since therapists were scarce due to the explosion of kids needing services, wait lists were the norm, and we fretted that our window of opportunity to make a positive impact was closing.

One night at a parent training session, the instructor told us we needed to approach Brady's treatment like we just bought a business. We were now the proud owners of a company that had employees (therapists and teachers), calendars, budgets, transportation needs, performance goals, and research/development. The only problem—we just bought a business in an industry we knew nothing about.

That analogy made sense to John and me because of our business backgrounds. We needed to learn about this company we just took over. So, John and I did what we both do best. I talked to doctors, therapists, moms, teachers, and tried to soak in as much as I could from the myriad of appointments I sat through with Brady. John read books. Lots of them. He went to the library, researched things online, watched YouTube videos, and compiled a list of activities designed to help with Brady's development. He created spreadsheets to keep track of our actions and Brady's therapies. To John, knowledge was power, and activity was the key to results.

We created a weekly newsletter called "Learning Objectives and Teaching Activities" that we updated and emailed every Sunday to our family, Brady's teachers, providers, and caregivers. Our goal was to create some consistency around the interactions with Brady so he could catch up to his peers. We couldn't parent him effectively on the fly, and we knew that anything we were encouraging him to do at home could be unraveled if it wasn't enforced throughout his day.

For instance, if we wanted Brady to speak in a normal voice, we couldn't respond when he used the squealing, screeching, high-pitched tone that nearly shattered glass. But, no matter how committed we were to that strategy at home, if he went to see his grandparents and they responded to his silly voice, he would keep using it.

Every Sunday night, John and I would review the notes from his teachers, therapists, and our own research, and would send out the newsletter. We included things we considered "wins"—like evaluations that showed improvement or interactions we noted with peers—but we were also very candid about the hard moments. While we didn't go into detail on each one, we thought it was important that the people closest to us understood exactly why their cooperation was so important.

John also created games for Brady that motivated him to learn. "Nanas in the Cupboard" was one of Brady's favorites. When he was about three, Brady's cousin Lexi gave him a small stuffed monkey for Christmas, and it became his constant companion. Brady wisely named the doll "Nanas" since monkeys eat bananas. By the time we realized that Brady had autism, Nanas had lived with us for almost a year, and he was already showing signs of how well Brady loved him. His fur was slightly matted, and the soft fabric around his face held scars from being dragged absentmindedly across the tile floors. A good mother probably would have hand-washed the doll on a regular basis to keep him sanitary, but it never crossed my mind to separate Brady and his best friend.

I wish I could remember how Nanas wound up in the cupboard the first time. I assume it was intentional, but it also could have been the result of lack of sleep or caffeine. When John found Nanas behind the door, tucked in next to the Goldfish crackers and cereal, he shouted in surprise and asked how in the world a monkey got in the cupboard! Brady cackled like it was the funniest thing he'd ever seen. From all the research he had done and parent training we had received, John knew he had motivational gold at his fingertips.

Almost every day, John would pick a skill that Brady needed to practice. If he completed the activity, John would stand up and wander into the kitchen murmuring to himself, "I sure am hungry! I think I'm gonna mosey on over to the cupboard to get some snacks!" Then he would open the door dramatically, pull out Nanas, and exclaim, "Wait a second, how did a monkey get in my cupboard???" Brady was usually so tickled he would continue with multiple iterations of the undesirable work just to get the few moments of joy when he was reunited with his monkey.

Playing on Brady's new love of superheroes, John even created a new dynamic duo to help him learn. "Ida B. Morfunn" was the evil supervillain who tried to steal Brady's attention and distract him from his task. "Seymore Gettindon" would battle Ida by blasting her with focus bombs to keep her frozen until Brady's task was complete.

John and I were constantly working to create forward momentum with a goal of steepening the slope of Brady's learning curve so he could catch up with his peers. John was the researcher and visionary, and I was the ground operations leader. Together, we gradually learned the business of caring for our son. But still, behind all the activity, I was haunted by the core belief that I was not equipped to be a special needs mom. I wasn't prepared for autism, I wasn't educated about autism, I wasn't enough for autism.

When we are called to a situation that is foreign to us, we will feel ill-equipped. And nothing we are called to, especially the hard things, will come with a quick start kit to give us everything we need to be awesome out of the gate. We won't feel equipped because we aren't equipped.

But here is the secret that I didn't understand at the time. We don't need to feel equipped to be effective. Our feelings don't drive results. Our actions do. All we need is a willingness to take the next step forward. We need to get up the next morning, read the next article, go to the next appointment, and talk to the next person. If we keep finding the next thing to do, even if it's a mistake, it is experience.

Just like we learned to keep Beagle Bailey from pooping on the carpet and attacking other dogs, we would learn to be the parents of this special boy that we were called to raise. And along the way, I would find that what I was lacking was not education, expertise, or experience. It was a relationship with the One who called me.

CHAPTER 6
ENSLAVED OR ENTRUSTED

While I have always called myself a Christian, it was more of a characteristic than a statement of relationship. Like I'm short, or blonde (with a little chemical help), or Irish. I went to church as a kid and had a few "God moments" at summer camp, so I believed in Jesus on some level. But church was just part of our weekly routine, not a chance to connect personally with our Creator.

When my family moved from Spokane, Washington, to Scottsdale, Arizona, in 1986, my parents started attending a large Presbyterian church about 20 minutes from our home. The pastor was from our old church in Spokane and looked so much like my dad that parishioners would frequently mix them up. Tom had a deep, powerful voice, and each Sunday, he would impart spiritual wisdom mixed with funny jokes and an understanding of scripture. But most of all he never, ever went over his allotted time, which I think my Dad appreciated the most.

As a teenager I was fairly disengaged from the church, although I loved going to the Christmas Eve services there. In addition to the huge organ, they always had a string quartet and sometimes a brass section as well. The large choir of older men and women wore traditional baby-blue satin robes with white sashes draped around their necks, and you could tell by the shape of their mouths as they sang that many were professionally trained. The finale of the indoor service was the "Hallelujah" chorus, and it always brought tears to my eyes, as did the a cappella version of "Silent Night" that closed the evening around the candlelit fountain.

When my parents decided to become formal members of the church, we learned that because I was 16, the church would require me to become a member on my own instead of through a family plan. It seems a little unfair in today's standards, considering kids in their late twenties can still attach themselves to their parents' health insurance. But I appreciated the nod to my near-adulthood, and agreed to meet with the youth pastor so he could guide me through the steps to be accepted into the church roster.

When I arrived at the church, I was led into Pastor Bob's office, where he asked me to sit on his couch. He turned toward his desk, picked up a yellow pad and a pen, and placed them in my lap. He told me he needed to make sure my spiritual knowledge was sufficient for the church to accept me as a member, so he needed me to write a page each on God, Jesus, the Holy Spirit, the Church, the Trinity, and Eternal Life. I looked at him incredulously but did not pick up the pen. I remember thinking there was no way this guy was going to make me sit there and write a six-page essay on a yellow pad. I was a busy high school junior with plenty of REAL homework, and if it didn't count for a grade, I wasn't doing it.

I put the pad and the pen back down on the coffee table, and as politely as I could muster, I said, "I'm not going to do that. If you have questions about my knowledge of faith, why don't you just ask me?" Fortunately, he agreed, and after about 30 minutes of questions, I passed the oral test. It was an homage to my Whitworth Presbyterian Sunday School teachers and to my ability to think on my feet. With the first hurdle cleared, there was just one more thing I had to do to be a member—get baptized.

My parents never baptized me as a baby, so the pastor scheduled the baptism for the next Sunday during the main church service.

Growing up Presbyterian, I had never watched anyone get baptized who counted their age in years instead of months, so it was awkward and slightly embarrassing for me to get up in front of the entire congregation and get a few drops of water placed on my head. Besides that, I have unruly curls, so when my mechanically straightened hair makes contact with water, my style tends to unravel into a mess reminiscent of Medusa. But, in the end, I wanted to please my parents and put the episode behind me, so I stood up in front of hundreds of strangers and was baptized with little fanfare or celebration. When I walked out of the church, I felt nothing but relief that the whole process was over.

In my twenties, I kept God at arm's length so as not to have Him cramp my party-girl style. I was living in Southern California at the beach with my college friends, and Sundays were mostly spent recovering from Saturday night instead of darkening the doorway of a church. However, when I learned one of my former youth pastors from Spokane was visiting a congregation in Riverside, about an hour away, I decided to take it easy on Saturday night so I could drive out to say hello.

Entering the small community sanctuary, I was uneasy, as if I were an intruder in someone else's home. I was a poser—a pretender who wasn't there for the right reasons. But the familiar combination of the music and the message quickly put me at ease. I lingered after the service and reminisced with my former mentor, and by the time I left, I felt ten pounds lighter. I had a sense of peace and contentment that stayed with me through the day. I convinced myself it was just because I'd been productive instead of laying on my couch watching reruns of *Beverly Hills, 90210.*

By the time I moved back to Arizona in 2002, my party habits were tamed, but I was still not willing to give up a Sunday morning for anything but a good cup of coffee, a long walk, or a workout at the gym. Then I met John in 2005. He lived about twenty miles away and had been attending a small community church service in a school gymnasium. He said he liked it because they let him bring his coffee to his seat. I quickly suggested all kinds of other activities we could pursue on Sunday mornings, and within a few weeks of meeting me, he never brought up going to church again. I used to joke that I corrupted him. Now, sadly, I know I did.

When John and I finally married and became parents, we figured it was time to plant some spiritual roots. Our motivation was to give Brady a good, moral upbringing, and we thought church was part of that equation. So, we agreed to start visiting churches of different denominations in our neighborhood. John's only rule was that the pastors could not wear robes, so that eliminated the Presbyterian church I was comfortable with.

The first church we tried was a non-denominational church about five minutes from our home. We dropped Brady at Sunday School and took it as a good sign that he didn't start screaming as we walked away.

When we entered the auditorium and saw the concert-style seating, audio-visual equipment, and drummer's box on stage, we hesitated for a moment. Neither of us had ever been to a church service like this before, but we found our seats and settled in. We rose to our feet with the rest of the congregation as the lights came down and the rock show began. The band was incredible, and I immediately found myself clapping to the beat and swaying to the harmonies. I was lost in the inspirational music until I noticed several members of the congregation lifting their hands in the air. That stopped me cold.

Was this some type of cult? Who does that? Why? Are they brainwashed, or groupies, or worse? I was relieved when the pastor came out and started the sermon, and I even overlooked the fact that he was wearing skinny jeans and a form-fitted hoodie. I figured if robes were out, I would have to get used to a hipster in the pulpit.

The topic of the message was the story of Joseph in the Bible. Joseph was not just the inspiration for a Broadway musical, but he did have a coat of many colors, and his brothers betrayed him and sold him into slavery. When the pastor directed our attention to the big screen behind the stage for a video clip that would illustrate his point, John and I were stunned when an episode of *Duck Dynasty* started to roll. Now mind you, it was a great sermon, and the TV show did highlight relevant brotherly interactions, but John and I just weren't ready for it. The drums, ducks, and demonstrative praise were a shock to our conservative systems, so while we enjoyed the day, we decided to move on.

We tried several other churches within our geographic radius, but they also became one-hit wonders in our search. In most cases, Brady was the determining factor. No matter how decorative the children's classrooms looked, how many toys they had, or how sweet the volunteers seemed, Brady would cast his "nay" vote by screaming for Mommy throughout the service. Rarely were John and I able to hear the end of a sermon because our claim check number would appear on the screen behind the pastor, along with a request that we pick up our child early.

Eventually we tired of the tour of churches. Instead, we often chose sleep over spiritual awakening on Sundays. Brady was wired with an internal alarm clock that was set for 4:30 a.m. Every. Single. Day. I woke up with him during the work week, and John and I tag-teamed the weekend days. Sunday was John's day to get up, and although I couldn't sleep late with the ruckus going on in the family room, I clung to my alone time, nestled snugly in bed. Once I was up and around, I was not inclined to put the effort into making myself ready to face the world with a shower and makeup.

John and I rationalized our laziness. Brady was attending a Lutheran preschool, so his weekly chapel classes and our occasional appearance at school performances and holidays probably provided enough religion for us to get by. The contemporary branch of the school's church, Megalife, even helped John and me get over our discomfort with modern services. The church founder was a former member of the heavy metal band Megadeath, who converted to Christianity years earlier. We liked the music, and we even started to appreciate the concert atmosphere and casual dress code, but we were still missing something we couldn't explain.

John suggested we should give the *Duck Dynasty* church another try now that we had acclimated to a contemporary worship format. I agreed. Megalife helped me make peace with people who worshiped with their hands raised to heaven. I understood it was a sign of surrender, of reverence, and of humility. I never told John, but I secretly wished I could be that free—to worship God with abandon, not worrying how it appeared to other rigid and self-conscious churchgoers like me. So, the next Sunday, we showed up at McDowell Church, keeping an open mind.

This time, almost two years after our first visit, something was different. The music was still stirring and hands were in the air, but that day, the sermon seemed to speak directly to my heart. This was the point in our autism journey with Brady that was the darkest for me. I was exhausted, frustrated, and frankly, mad at God for taking my perfectly good life plan and throwing a stick in my wheel. But the pastor spoke to my brokenness, and I left wondering if God had sent that message just for me.

I realize now He had. It's a phenomenon of faith that we will never fully understand, and we should never ignore. God somehow makes us hear what he wants to tell us, whether through a pastor, a friend, or even an acquaintance on the street. Just like the gradual process the Holy Spirit used to bring us awareness of Brady's autism, He used the pastor's words to draw me closer. So, I went back the next Sunday and the next, and the same thing happened each week.

One Sunday in particular, the band performed a song called "No Longer Slaves." It hit me between the eyes—that's what I felt like. A slave. I was a slave to therapies, to self-imposed isolation, to the next tantrum that may be around the corner. But mostly, I was a slave to fear. Fear of what Brady's future would look like, fear that the rest of my life was going to be dictated by Brady's needs, fear that I would never feel in control again.

I wept as the chorus repeated, "I'm no longer a slave to fear. I am a child of God." It gave me hope and exposed the destructive mindset I was stuck in. I had a beautiful, funny, healthy child whose brain worked a little differently. I was not *enslaved*. I was *entrusted*. God believed that my son needed to be part of the world, and He picked me to be Brady's mom. He trusted me to be Brady's mom.

To what have you been entrusted? What seems like a burden to you today but could be recharacterized as a blessing when you decide you are not a slave to it? The circumstances of your life do not determine your ability to experience joy and fulfillment. You do. I'm not saying that you should be oblivious to pain during really hard times in your life. We are all human, and there will be times when we will feel overwhelmed and sad. But instead of focusing on the circumstance, try focusing on what God is helping you learn or what he is equipping you for. Sometimes, pain has a purpose.

My pain was real, but it was also self-induced. I was clinging desperately to my broken plan, unwilling to accept that maybe, just maybe, God's plan was better. I was sacrificing the joy I had in front of me for the bitterness of misplaced entitlement to a life that never belonged to me. I was in chains of my own making, refusing to recognize that what I thought was holding me back was really leading me to a new purpose.

You may be fortunate to have known the love of Christ your whole life, but if not, I want to encourage you that finding faith usually doesn't come in a bolt of lightning. Faith isn't won in a race, and it is almost never a straight line from point A to point B. If you don't have a relationship with God yet, I hope my sharing the long, winding road I traveled encourages you that your path, with all the twists, turns, and potholes, is equipping you for the mission to which you have been entrusted.

I finally felt like the wall preventing me from stepping fully into faith was beginning to crumble, but I needed more. The sermons and songs only whet my appetite to dig deeper, and I pondered my next step.

CHAPTER 7
THE MASTERPiECE

Just as I was starting to consider the possibility of truly leaning into faith, God decided to give me a push. I received an email from McDowell announcing the next session of Women's Bible Study. It didn't seem like something I would be even remotely interested in. The term "Bible Study" brought up mental images of old silver-haired ladies rocking in chairs by a fire, reading the Bible with colorful homemade quilts covering their legs. In fact, a couple of years earlier, when a "young" (translation = my age) neighbor friend of mine mentioned she was going to a weekly Bible study, I was taken aback. I even thought it was weird.

But the Holy Spirit had planted the seed, and as he tends to do with his divine nudges, he continued to apply increasing force until I decided I should check it out.

I won't lie; walking into my first Bible Study was frightening. I felt like a kindergartener walking into a high school physics class. But as I looked around, I didn't see frail old ladies whispering quietly in their rocking chairs. I saw dozens of women of all ages having deep conversations, laughing, and hugging each other. It seemed promising, and it did not disappoint. These ladies were in love with Jesus, and it made me want to love Him too. I found myself immediately hooked on the fellowship, teaching, and even the homework, which challenged me to apply scripture to my own life.

One night, after Brady went to bed, I settled in on the couch with my Bible, study book, and pen. John liked to go into our bedroom to read, so I had the family room to myself, with the exception of our beagle, Bailey, who was curled up on the floor below me in the corner of the sectional.

As most studies do, the author asked us to read a few verses of the Bible. That night, this is what I read: *As he (Jesus) went along, he saw a man blind from birth. His disciples asked him, "Rabbi, who sinned, this man or his parents, that he was born blind?" "Neither this man nor his parents sinned," said Jesus, "but this happened so that the works of God might be displayed in him."* (John 9:1-3 NIV)

I stopped reading and put the book down for a moment. My breath caught in my chest. I was almost afraid to keep going because my soul stirred with that feeling from Sunday morning sermons that God was speaking right to me. Tentatively, like it might jump out and bite me, I picked up the Bible and read the passage again, and again. Then, I felt a surge of pressure in my head and in my heart, and my vision blurred from the tears gathering in my eyelids.

My brain was spinning, desperately trying to accept what I read. Could it be true? I believed that Brady had not sinned. He was a child and could not control the way his brain worked. But what about me? Could I believe that it was not my sin that caused his autism? Could I let go of the shame and guilt? Could I look past the things that make Brady different so I could see that God made him the way he is on purpose, for a purpose?

There was so much packed into those few sentences of scripture. I related to the blind man's parents. I encountered similar judgment from some parents at Brady's school. Even the disciples assumed that the blind man's condition was due to sin, and they overlooked the worth of the man himself. But Jesus saw him for who he really was and what he could do—glorify God. This was a revelation of identity and a wake-up call for me. I needed to stop looking in the carnival mirror held by the rest of the world, which showed us bent, disfigured, and broken, and see Brady how God did. Perfectly purposeful.

If you are looking in that same carnival mirror, step away now. The image is distorted. It's not you. Start seeing yourself through the eyes of the God who created you to bring glory to His name.

That is your purpose. That is Brady's purpose too. When I stopped focusing on what was different, hard, and unfair, I started to see the beauty and potential of what Brady could do, not *despite* how his brain works . . . but *because* of it.

Coming to Jesus is not a magic elixir for what the world dishes out. However, it can change your perspective. It gives you a handhold that you can reach for when you start to fall. It gives you identity as a child of the Creator of the world, who was created for a special purpose that no one else could accomplish but you. That revelation had eluded me most of my life.

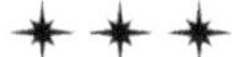

When I was in my early twenties, my boss asked me to attend a big charity dinner with him at the Forum near downtown Los Angeles. It was a black-tie event featuring Michael Eisner, then the CEO of Disney, as the keynote speaker. I was excited about the opportunity to get a free, fancy meal and maybe even see some famous people. I didn't own a formal dress, nor could I afford to buy one. Luckily, my roommate, Carolyn, had a little black Armani dress she was willing to lend. When I say "little" black dress, it was just that. Short. But beggars can't be choosers, and it was free, so I went with it.

After work that day, my boss and I changed into our formalwear at the office and he drove us downtown. We parked by an open door just a few feet from the car, got out and headed down a bright, narrow hallway, at least the length of a football field. The whole way I was fidgeting with my dress to get every spare inch of length to cover my bare legs. We finally came to a plain metal door and walked through it into a warmly lit room with several other well-dressed couples drinking champagne and chatting softly. I looked around and realized that Michael Eisner was right in front of me. Wow! My boss must have purchased a VIP ticket for this event, and we had backstage access for a meet and greet!

Before I had a chance to introduce myself, one of the men in tuxedos told us to line up. My boss grabbed my arm and gently led me to my place in line as confusion overtook me. Why did we have to line up to go into the event? I didn't get to ask because the line started moving briskly back out into the hallway, and after a couple more turns, we opened a door with nothing but blackness behind it. That's when my boss leaned down and whispered, "OK, after the host introduces us, just walk down the stairs to the table and take the seat next to me." *Wait, what? Introduce us? To whom?* Suddenly, my eyes started to adjust to the darkness, and around a thick velvet curtain, I could see a stage. Beyond it was a sea of richly adorned circular tables with about a thousand people in tuxedos and sparkly dresses chatting and enjoying their salads.

The reality of what was about to happen hit me. My boss and I weren't guests at this event. We were at the head table. He was well-known in California politics, so it made sense that he was given a place of honor, but why didn't he tell me I was going to be on display, too? I was going to have to walk out on that stage in my too-short dress and scuffed-up work heels with my boss, who was 40 years older than me, and then I would have to navigate down ten narrow steps to the table without falling on my face, flashing the elite men and women of Los Angeles.

The lights hit the stage, and the emcee welcomed and thanked the crowd for their attendance. Then, he started the introductions. First was the Lieutenant Governor and his wife, then a famous author and her husband, and then it was our turn.

The host read the list of public service positions held by my boss, and then after announcing his full name, he tagged on ". . . and guest." Apparently, that was me. The crowd started to applaud politely as I walked past the curtains to take in the full view of the arena. I looked out at all the faces. It may have been my imagination, but I swear I saw wide eyes and heard audible gasps and whispers as this dignitary held his arm for the blonde, inappropriately dressed date not important enough to have her own name.

Thankfully, the story doesn't end with me doing a triple lindy down the stairs. I had an uneventful descent to the table and was finally able to relax and enjoy the rest of the evening with the celebrities, including Mr. Eisner, who took pity on the blonde "nobody" at their table.

Walking across that stage, I was *exposed* and *unseen* at the same time. It may sound like an oxymoron, but that's how I often felt as the mother of a child with autism. Public meltdowns were an obvious source of scrutiny without understanding. But the feeling also crept in as I watched a group of other moms whisper while looking in my direction. Or during meetings with the school administrators about the support Brady needed. Or at Cub Scout meetings when Brady couldn't stay with the group or follow directions. Whether it was real or perceived, I felt other parents, teachers, or even random bystanders judging our worth. But they had no idea who we were and what we were going through.

If you feel that way too, please reread John 9. Jesus left no doubt that the blind man's life and his parents' lives were filled with God-given purpose and potential. So is yours. The key is to get from feeling exposed and unseen, to safe and seen.

To do that, we must focus on this truth. Our gifts, talents, failures, and flaws are all part of a custom package God designed so that we could accomplish His will during our lifetime. He gave us all the tools, but it's up to us to use them. God doesn't make mistakes. Ever. Sometimes, it's hard for me to remember, especially when I wish I was four inches taller with a faster metabolism, but it's true. Our identity doesn't come from family, friends, or Instagram—it comes from God. John 9 is proof of that.

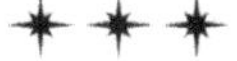

The author of Hebrews tells us that the Word of God is alive and active, and that night on my couch, it jumped out and grabbed me by my earlobes. I felt lighter and more peaceful knowing God wasn't punishing me and that He had great plans for Brady. But I was not the one dealing with a brain that functioned differently. Brady was. Things were hard for him, and when the time came for him to know about autism and ADHD, I didn't want him to use his diagnosis as an excuse or to wear it like a suit of armor, protecting him from experiences that would help him reach his potential.

It was just before Brady started second grade that John and I decided to tell him that he had autism and ADHD. He would be attending a school with other kids with diagnoses like his, and we wanted him to be prepared. I sat down at the computer to pull everything together. I wanted to give him the facts about how his brain works, but I also wanted to make him proud of who he is. I wanted him to understand why he has challenges but know that any challenge can be overcome with hard work. I wanted to validate his difficulties but fill him with hope for his future.

I collected clinical research, notes, and fun kid-centered videos, but still, something was missing. I wanted to make sure his identity was not centered on autism. I needed to prove to Brady he was wonderfully made, exactly as he is, for a purpose. Fortunately, the Holy Spirit took over the creative writing at that point, and together, we penned this poem.

Before I held you in my arms, I prayed to God above,
To bless you with a healthy body and sweet heart full of love.
The Good Lord heard my prayers but gave you so much more,
A rare collection of unique gifts and personality galore!

Your memory, sense of humor, and creative talents abound,
Your intelligence and happy nature bring smiles to all around.
I know there are some things in life that are hard for you to do,
But your gifts AND your struggles are part of God's plan for you.

You love your couch for squeezing and "squishes" help your mood,
You are not a fan of hand dryers, the blender, or hot food.
Sometimes, it's hard to make new friends, focusing is tough,
Unless it's something you enjoy—then you can't get enough!

All these things about you come from differences in your brain.
But things that don't come naturally we can work on to retrain.
There is no achievement you can't reach, no obstacle too high,
Your life can be what you design, dream big and always try.

So many people love you and want to help you on your way,
You've worked so hard and we can see the progress every day.
Your special brain has made you like no other from the start,
We wouldn't want you any different—you are God's work of art.

When I finished explaining everything to Brady, I read the

poem. Then, I gave him space to respond. In the moments of silence, I tried to read his expression. I admit I had visions in my head of our tearful embrace, Brady showering me with gratitude for finally helping him understand his worth. Before you grab your tissues for the Hallmark moment you are expecting, Brady just said, "OK. Can I have some screen time now?" Turns out autistic elementary schoolers aren't wired for emotional storybook endings. That's how God made him. But ever since, we have done our best to reinforce his worth, his purpose, and his potential. To prove to Brady his identity is rooted in God's plan.

I know we haven't met, but there is one thing I know for sure. God made you, your child, and everyone around you just right. Under His love and protection, you are safe and seen, not exposed and unseen. He made you for a purpose, and it doesn't have to be some grandiose accomplishment the whole world sees. You don't have to write a book or start a global non-profit. Your purpose may be to encourage someone, to hire someone, to birth someone, or to love someone. Your purpose may be to build something, write something, say something, or create something. If you find your identity in who God made you to be, you will bring glory to Him. Just like Brady, you are God's work of art.

PART 2:

ADAPTiNG

"The best thing about the future is that it comes only one day at a time."
—Abraham Lincoln

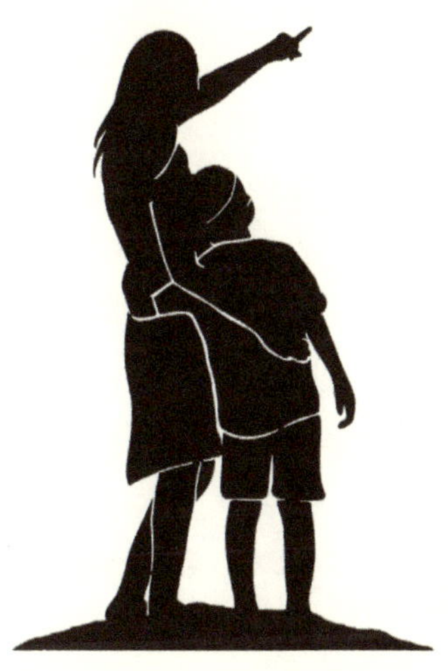

CHAPTER 8
MULTiPLY

I am a social person, and I've never been shy. On more than one occasion, I have been known to confidently approach "famous" people—CEOs, actors, or sports figures—holding out my hand for a shake as if we were long-lost friends, much to the horror of my real friends. My outgoing nature has helped me in many areas of my life. But in all honesty, I'm afraid the root of my perkiness is an underlying desire to please others and, dare I say it, impress them. I like putting my best foot forward, even if my foot just stepped in doggie doo.

After my first knee surgery, I woke up from the anesthesia violently ill and in unbearable pain. I was taking turns sobbing and vomiting into a dish by the bed as the nurses tried to figure out what was wrong. Suddenly I got a clear look at the crowd around my bed and noticed one of the nurses was a client of mine. I immediately stopped crying, tried to sit up, smile, and offer a casual greeting as though she had just walked into my office for a portfolio review. She giggled and reminded me I was in her office, and I didn't have to pretend everything was okay. Thank goodness, but it still didn't sit well with me that she saw me at my worst.

When John and I became parents, I was fully prepared to be the best mom ever, an example to new parents everywhere of poise, patience, and perfection. Sadly, I realized very early on I was not on track to win the prize, but it didn't stop me from trying to appear as though I was still in the running.

The more Brady's behaviors emerged at school or out in public, the harder it was to play the part. He would run away at parties or ignore the other kids. We would go to restaurants or entertainment venues, and he would melt down. Our decision to only tell our closest friends, family, and teachers about his diagnosis put up an invisible wall. Everyone on the other side of the wall got a scripted response if they asked about his behavior or developmental progress, and then we would make a quick exit. It wasn't quite a lie, but it felt like one.

Our friends and family who knew the truth about Brady were incredibly supportive, but we even held back from them, not wanting to divulge the nitty-gritty of our imperfect life. My friends with kids were excited to share all the milestones their children were hitting, as they should have been. But every text or post about their successes felt like our failures. We felt different. We felt flawed. We felt alone.

Sometimes, our challenges make us feel like we are in exile. Forced to be somewhere we don't want to be. Separated from a life we once knew. Isolated by the misguided notion that no one understands or has survived a situation like ours. Here's the thing—you are not alone in feeling alone! Don't let the lie that your struggle is completely unique, prevent you from seeking community.

Exile is a repeated theme in the Bible, and God gives us an instruction book to handle it. When the Israelites were in Babylon, they lost everything they held dear. Their homes, their temple, their freedom, their entire way of life. But God didn't want them to wallow in their separation. And God doesn't want us to steep in the disappointment and discouragement of our perceived exile either. Even in tough times, he wants us to thrive as he works His plan for our good. He encouraged His people to build houses, plant gardens, and multiply. Multiply, in its very definition, requires more than one. You need to find community.

While John and I kept our circle small, I did disclose Brady's diagnosis to my business partner, Renee, and my close friend, Lisa. Surprisingly, Renee and Lisa both had friends with boys on the spectrum. They offered to share my contact information, and

I enthusiastically agreed. These women called me within the same day and spent more than an hour on the phone listening to me. They answered my rapid-fire questions and provided validation of our concerns. I took pages of notes as we discussed the similarities and differences between Brady and their sons. I had never met these women, yet they dedicated their time and valuable perspective as parents who were much further down the autism road than I.

This was weeks before we even had a formal diagnosis. I was just dipping my toe in the shallow end of autism, and I was all about the information. Just the facts, ma'am. I wasn't looking for friends; I needed guidance. At the end of each conversation I thanked the women profusely, hung up, and focused my attention and energy on motoring full speed ahead.

It only took a few months of living the life of an autism mom before exhaustion and loneliness set in. I realized this was a long haul and not a short sprint, and maintaining our public façade that everything was okay was starting to wear on me.

One afternoon I was at occupational therapy with Brady, and his provider gave me a pink sticky note with the name "Amy" and a phone number. Amy was a mom of another patient, a boy about Brady's age with autism. Amy told the OT to give her number out to any new family that started therapy there. She wanted to be a resource to parents standing at the trailhead of the long hike of autism treatment.

I waited a few days to call. For some reason I felt awkward, and my formerly extroverted self was hesitant to call a stranger. But I also didn't want to go to Brady's next OT session and report that I had failed to follow instructions, (I'm a people pleaser, remember?) so I dialed her number, expecting a voicemail.

Amy answered, which surprised me, but I explained why I was calling, and she sounded pleased that I had reached out. We discussed our boys' ages, where they were going to school, and where we lived, and then Amy invited me to join her and a few other moms for coffee later that week.

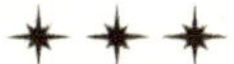

It poured down rain that morning. If you live in Arizona, morning rain storms don't happen very often, and neither our roads nor our drivers are well equipped for navigating the streets. In fact, many of us sunshine dwellers will cancel plans outside the house on rainy days because we don't own rain boots and umbrellas. You think I'm exaggerating, but we have a Wicked-Witch-of-the-West-level aversion to rain here. I considered sending a text that I couldn't make it, knowing the rain was a semi-valid excuse, but decided to venture out anyway. Again, the people pleaser in me didn't want to be labeled a flake, and that overrode my newfound social anxiety.

I ran into the grocery store with my coat extended over my head, trying to keep my naturally curly hair from the rain. I found the coffee shop, and Amy and her friends were already at the table. I don't know why it surprised me that they were all pretty and stylish. I guess I thought everyone in my situation should look like I felt—like the Hunchback of Notre Dame.

The women greeted me warmly, and within minutes of sitting down, I realized the dynamic of this group was different. Way different. They talked about ABA (Applied Behavior Analysis), speech, occupational therapy, physical therapy, and social skills groups. I told them about Brady's obsession with *Wiggles* DVD covers, and they all laughed knowingly and shared similar stories from their family. They talked about struggles with the school district, getting access to providers, and feeding their picky eaters. We spoke freely with no filter about parenting our special kids, the good, the bad, and the messy. With this group, I could drop the tap dance. It was as if I had been living the last year in a country where no one spoke English, and I finally found someone who spoke my language. Not long into the conversation, I was crying tears of joy and relief—I wasn't alone anymore.

I was still in exile, but I was not the only one living here. Over the years, this group supported each other through school changes, social challenges, medication decisions, and therapy schedules. We met other moms in clinic waiting rooms and summer camps for special kids and invited them to join us. We empathized with each other when things went poorly and celebrated the smallest victory. Even as schedules got more challenging and we couldn't meet as often, we were still just a phone call or text away for a question or concern.

In community with each other, we could shed the suit of armor we wore with the rest of the world and strip down to our authentic selves. We were free from judgment from those who dwelled outside the walls of autism, and we built our houses, planted our gardens, and multiplied.

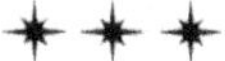

I believe God gives us a special kind of radar that allows us to recognize others who are going through similar situations in life. As the years passed, and I became more comfortable talking about Brady's diagnosis, I began to connect with other concerned moms at church, Brady's school, the grocery store checkout line, pretty much everywhere I found people. I've been contacted by multiple moms who got my number from a friend or therapist. Now, I am the one giving a stranger an hour of my time to meet an immediate need. I've also had dozens of coffee meetings, lunches, and parking lot conversations with worried parents. Sometimes, our situations were completely different, but at least we spoke the same language.

I also found we understood each other regardless of the specific diagnosis or lack thereof. The kids at the center of my conversations had a myriad of neurological differences other than autism, such as ADHD, anxiety, sensory processing disorder, dyslexia, or obsessive-compulsive disorder. Even if the parent had not pursued an evaluation yet, there was one common thread: all these children looked just like every other child, but behaviors at home, at school, and in the community indicated a difference in the way the child received information.

In 2018, at the prompting of a woman in my Bible Study, I started writing about some of the early days of our awareness of Brady's autism. I mostly wrote a narrative of the hard stuff, a brain dump of the scenes that weren't already clouded by a dense fog in my mind. I thought our story might encourage another family looking for community in exile.

As I documented the painful memories, God gave me the acronym KIND—Kids with Invisible Neurological Differences. The name fit Brady and just about every other child whose parents had come to me for support. KIND kids look like every other kid, but because of the way their brains are wired, they react and impact the world in a way that is unfamiliar to teachers, peers, and neighbors.

If you have been through a tough time, God wants you to use what you learned to help others in the same situation. In 2 Corinthians, Paul tells us that God comforts us so we can comfort others. You don't need to impart wisdom and instruction. You don't need to fix them. You just need to be present and prove that they are not alone. That is the heart behind KIND Families.

In a recent church service, our pastor told a story about Moses that struck a chord with me. Moses was chosen by God to lead His people, the Israelites, out of slavery in Egypt. After they escaped from the Egyptian army through the parting of the Red Sea, the Israelites wandered in the desert for decades, with Moses as their guide, on their way to the promised land.

One day, Moses ordered Joshua to take some men to fight an enemy in a valley below. Moses stood on a hill overseeing the battle. As long as he held the staff of God over his head, the Israelites would start to win the battle. But, if he dropped his arms, the enemy would start to overtake them.

I don't know how heavy the staff was, but I bet no amount of Pilates can prepare your biceps, triceps, and traps for holding a large wooden tree above you for the length of a military offensive. Understandably, Moses got to a point where he physically couldn't hold the staff up any longer. That's when his brother Aaron and his friend Hur stepped in. They brought a stone for Moses to sit on, and then they held his arms up for him. The Israelites won the battle, and Moses got a hot bath and a neck massage—at least, I hope he did.

Aaron and Hur epitomized the power of friendship, support, and community. If Moses failed, people would have died. But the weight of the responsibility was overwhelming, and Moses grew weary. Aaron and Hur recognized their friend's fatigue, understood the importance of his mission, and stepped in to help.

But why didn't Aaron and Hur just take the staff out of Moses's hands and hold it for him? That would have made more sense to me. They could just take turns holding the staff, passing it off when one became tired. Even better, two men could hold each end of the staff with Moses in the middle.

Instead, Aaron and Hur supported Moses while he held on to the staff. They didn't remove the burden. They couldn't—the burden wasn't theirs to bear. God placed the responsibility of victory in the battle on Moses alone. But when fatigue set in, Aaron and Hur surrounded Moses and found a way to lighten his load.

Are you carrying a heavy weight? Is the pressure getting tougher and tougher to sustain yourself? Unfortunately, your problem is not like a baton in a relay race. You can't pass it off to a teammate and watch her run around the track to the finish line. Your challenge may be more like a marathon, and no one else is equipped to hold the baton. But you don't have to run alone.

I am so grateful to Amy for inviting me into her community, but even if you haven't found a personal connection, there are online groups and counselors who can speak your language. Search Facebook or Instagram for whatever situation is pressing you into isolation, and I bet there is a group you can join that can relate. If you know or love a KIND kid, join the KIND Families Community.

Then, when you have a little road behind you, make yourself available to someone who could use your support and wisdom to navigate their own path. You don't have to be an expert or offer solutions, just share your story and your shoulder. Remember how you felt when you were at square one. What would have fed you during that time? Feed others what you hungered for. Your presence and perspective may be just what someone needs to learn to build, plant, and multiply—in community.

CHAPTER 9
SEARCHiNG FOR MRS. MUMBLES

When I was a kid, school choice had not been invented yet. At least not in Spokane, Washington. We simply attended the public school that was closest to our house. Period. I had limited awareness of any alternative to the public schools. Private schools conjured up mental images of wealthy, well-mannered kids in uniforms with lots of plaid and gold emblems—like the TV show *Silver Spoons*.

I was pregnant with Brady when John and I bought our first house together, and we felt like geniuses. The neighborhood was within walking or bike riding distance from the local public elementary, middle, and high school. Think of all the gas we would save! Think of all the time not wasted in a daily commute!

Preschool snuck up on me, though. I missed the memo that in Scottsdale, to enroll your kid in preschool, you must start researching the options twelve months in advance. Since Brady was born, I had managed my consulting business with babysitting help from my family, and juggled emails and calls during naps. I looked forward to Brady starting preschool so I could have a few hours per week of pre-planned work/private time. I figured (mistakenly) that I could start looking for a preschool a few months before the school year started. I was jolted into reality when another mommy in my Little Gym class asked where I was sending Brady for preschool. I replied casually, "I don't know—I'll probably start looking in the spring."

The woman looked at me with a combination of pity and horror. Didn't I know that registration started last month? No, I did not. Most schools already have waiting lists! For preschool??? Seriously?? Panic set in. I ran home, blew up the internet and the phone, and set out on a turbo-charged tour of preschools in the area. I was determined to rectify my error and secure my two-year-old a spot at the most prestigious preschool in town.

I quickly narrowed my search and set my sights on a Christian preschool recommended by my horrified Little Gym classmate. I had not discovered my faith yet, but I still wanted Brady to have a spiritual foundation, and I was woefully lacking in the necessary skills to teach him.

All the criteria boxes were checked. The school was close to home, the teachers were lovely, and it just felt right. I wasn't too concerned with curriculum, Brady was only two after all, but they had a pet chinchilla named Mrs. Mumbles and the cuteness factor was just too much to bear.

All that was left was to fill out the application and wait for school to start. Or so I thought. Turns out lots of other moms with future two-year-old prodigies were just as enchanted by Mrs. Mumbles, and there were going to be more applicants than spaces. Plus, families with kids already at the school and members of the church got priority, so according to our sources, there were only five or six spots open for new kiddos. How could we get to the top of the list? Fortunately, the school had a first come, first served system that opened for new families the following week.

Registration started at 8:00 a.m., and the only way to be at the front of the line was to get there early. Really early. We heard rumors that the year before parents showed up at 4:00 a.m. to claim a spot. Yep—4:00 a.m. Ridiculous, I know. I was not that parent, right? Wrong again.

It was a cold January morning with freezing temperatures the day John and I rolled out of bed at 3:00 a.m. to secure our son's educational future. We bundled up and drove to the school with lawn chairs, coffee mugs, blankets, and movies downloaded on the iPad. We figured we would be first in line. However, when we got to the parking lot, we were dismayed to see that we were not the first family in line. We weren't even the seventh family in line. So, while we felt crazy for getting up in the middle of the night to sit in the dark to get our toddler into preschool, we took some comfort in the fact that there were a few other families even more demented than we were.

It took several weeks to find out that we did get a spot for Brady, and we celebrated like we won the lottery. The preschool fed into a primary school on another campus that went through eighth grade. It wasn't walking distance to our house like the public school trifecta, but it was still a short drive. And after all that effort to get Brady's foot in the door, we were never leaving. At least, that was the plan.

A year later, when the autism diagnosis came, the preschool responded with love, acceptance, and nearly unlimited willingness to help. They allowed us to place a full-time aide in Brady's classroom to help with task completion and social situations, and they gave us access to a speech pathologist who agreed to meet with Brady before school several days per week. They loved Brady, so we loved them.

Brady's doctors told us it was best to keep him in a mainstream classroom so his peers could model appropriate behaviors, and that became paramount to us, especially after the experience with the public developmental school. We thought we were safe.

Then came kindergarten.

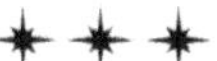

We got the first call right before Thanksgiving. John and I were asked to meet with the kindergarten teacher and the elementary school principal, with no indication of the reason for the discussion. At the meeting, we were shocked to learn that other parents had started complaining about the presence of kids like Brady on campus. There were two other children with autism in Brady's class of twenty, and some parents were concerned the school was more focused on special needs than academic excellence.

The message was loud and clear. Brady was welcome to keep his aide in the classroom through the end of kindergarten, but he would have to operate independently in first grade. We were stunned and scared—but weren't ready to jump ship yet.

We found a transformative behavioral therapist who, over several months, helped us wean Brady off the direct support he received from the aide. Miss Mckenzie created simple processes the teachers could use to keep Brady on task, and the school agreed Mckenzie could observe the class a couple of times a month to tweak the program if needed.

We were so proud that Brady was able to be independent in the classroom, and his first-grade teacher, who also had a daughter with developmental challenges, was Brady's biggest cheerleader.

Again, we breathed a sigh of relief. With the simple system the teacher administered, Brady was able to keep up academically. He also seemed to be doing well with the other neurotypical kids in his class. Having known Brady since preschool, his classmates accepted him. They knew he had some peculiarities, but they were very patient and inclusive with him.

When the school board brought in a new principal right before Christmas, I was fairly calm about it, even hopeful that maybe it would be a good thing for our family and the school. Until I got the email requesting another meeting to talk about Brady's enrollment for second grade. Here we go again.

I couldn't imagine how the administration could have a problem with Brady at this point. He was operating independently in class. His teacher was successfully running the prompting program with the help of one or two monthly visits from the lead therapist who adjusted the program as needed. In addition, a speech pathologist joined Brady for lunch and recess three days per week to help with social interactions with the other kids. He was by far the best reader in the class and stood out from his classmates in every area but math. Still, the writing was on the wall.

John wasn't available to go with me to meet with the principal, so I was on my own. I knew I had to keep my emotions in check, so before the meeting, I sat in my car in the parking lot and prayed that God would give me composure and the right words to have a productive conversation. I had heard that God can give you peace beyond your understanding, and I was in desperate need of peace. I am not a big crier, but ugly tears had a nasty habit of escaping at the most inopportune times. Usually when I was confronting a boss or an ex-boyfriend. Or my son's new principal.

I was right about the purpose of the meeting. He brushed through the pleasantries quickly and dropped the bomb that if Brady was going to attend second grade at the school, he would have to do so with zero accommodations, no prompting program, and no visits or recommendations from therapists. Apparently, complaints had resurfaced from other parents who were concerned the school was becoming known as a "special needs" school. The principal agreed, and his opinion was that Brady and the other kids with similar conditions were a distraction to teachers and other students.

As I listened, even though I was prepared for the direction of the conversation, it was like I was watching the dialogue as a passive observer. It was crazy to me that an educator of a Christian school with a motto that included being "Christ-like" would do something so blatantly contrary to what Jesus would do. He was basically expelling us, removing Brady from the only school he had known since he was two years old, and there was nothing we could do about it. Our choice—set Brady up to fail or leave. It was straightforward and perfectly legal. As a private school that did not take government funds, they didn't have to accommodate my son. I could feel my face getting hot and my pulse starting to race. I closed my eyes briefly and appealed to God to keep the tears from flowing. This man didn't deserve my tears.

My prayers were answered as I could palpably feel the peace that I prayed for lay on me like a warm blanket. I took a deep breath, and when I exhaled I did not cry. I steadied my voice. I very calmly told him I disagreed, that I believed his stance was not Christ-like, and I told him we would start looking for a new school.

We visited other Christian schools in the area, but they were all so large we were afraid Brady would be lost. There were Montessori schools nearby, but they lacked the kind of structure we knew Brady needed. Our experience with the public school system did not give us confidence that Brady's needs would be met, and the charter schools were too academically demanding.

That left one option: Lexis Preparatory, a small private school about five minutes from our home, which specialized in helping kids with learning differences.

The geography could not have been better, and based on my preschool requirements, it would have been perfect if they had a furry rodent as their mascot. But still, I resisted. I was so adamant that I wanted him in a mainstream classroom. I told myself it was because the doctors said he needed neurotypical models, but deep down, I knew that wasn't the reason. I told myself he needed to be in a Christian environment, even though we had come from one that was far from Christ-like.

No, I was clinging to my original plan. The plan that didn't include autism. The plan that gave me the school experience I dreamed about as a new mom. But that plan was not what Brady needed, and I had to let it go.

I finally agreed to take a tour of Lexis, and within minutes of talking to the lower school principal, I knew it was what Brady needed. The classes were very small, with individualized curriculums for each child, constant social skills and executive function training, and detailed performance tracking. John and I decided it was our best option. At least for now.

The time Brady spent at his new school was the most impactful of any of the other treatments and therapies we tried. He started to excel academically, make friends, and manage activities of daily life with a trajectory that was finally helping him catch up with his peers. In a way, I am grateful to his old school for pushing me out of the boat because otherwise, I would not have made the leap on my own.

I'd love to tell you that Brady still attends Lexis, but after two years, the Covid shutdown forced the school to close. We were devastated, but once again, God was faithful in leading us to a school that provided a temporary landing place, another specialty school about twenty miles away. I lamented the two hours a day in the car, but what I lost in gas money and time I gained in a newfound love of podcasts.

The fifth grade took us to another small Christian school with a heart for kids who learn differently. Brady was successful back in a mainstream classroom, building on the foundational skills he gathered at his last two stops. He made friends and participated in sports and student council, but after three years, we are once again on the move.

If there is one constant, it's change. We have learned as Brady grows his needs will shift, and we must adapt to meet him. Brady is crushing it academically now but struggling socially in the minefield of middle school. Today, my top priority is to protect his heart. Tomorrow, my priorities may change. My new plan is to scrap my old plan and leave the planning to God.

I have a very smart friend named Lori Taylor who started an organization called "Thriving in Between". She uses an analogy to describe our hesitance to let go. Imagine you are holding onto a rope. You grip the rope tightly because it was once your lifeline. But when it's time to reach for something new, if you don't loosen your grip on the old rope, you'll get a painful burn.

I had to learn to let go of the rope that was my naive expectation about stability in Brady's schooling. Instead of clinging desperately to a mainstream class, a specialty environment, or a Christian school with Mrs. Mumbles as the mascot, I need to be vigilantly searching for rope burns on my left hand and a new rope to grab with my right. When it comes to Brady's education, I'm like Tarzan swinging through the jungle.

Is there something you are struggling to release in your life? When you feel like you can't hold on anymore, that is probably the time to loosen your grip, turn around, and start reaching for what God has in store.

CHAPTER 10
THE iNViSiBiLiTY CLOAK

Brady has always been a voracious reader, something I consider an answered prayer. I had him later in life, so I learned from my friends who had children before me which activities were the easiest to deliver as a parent, and when I was pregnant, I guided my requests to God accordingly.

Basketball would be okay—it was usually indoors with air conditioning, but John and I weren't exactly blessed in the height department, so we knew that was a longshot. Baseball was a maybe—the games were outside, but the travel requirements seemed reasonable, and the games weren't as long. Soccer was a hard no. I watched my friends spend their entire weekends traversing the four corners of the state for soccer tournaments, and it seemed tortuous to me. First, I don't like soccer. Second, the meets were always played in the hottest parts of the year, so they would spend hours in lawn chairs in the blazing sun watching the kids run back and forth on the grass.

God took my requests seriously, and for the first decade of Brady's life he had absolutely no interest in anything that involved a ball, running, or sweat. Television and tablet screens were his favorite, but books were a close second. I read to him every night, and as his vocabulary increased, his desire for more intricate plotlines followed. We read every book in the *Magic Treehouse* series, the *Kingdom of Wrenly* stories, the *Narnia* books, and finally he asked to read the series his Auntie Kimberly had been promoting his whole life: *Harry Potter*.

If you are not familiar with the *Harry Potter* series, there are seven books, and in combination they have over 4,200 pages. Brady was only eight at the time, so I read a few chapters out loud to him before bedtime each night. Since I had never read the series, I relied on Auntie Kimberly to warn me when we were approaching an intense or scary scene, and I would summarize it without the details. We rarely missed a night of reading, and it took us almost a year to complete. Since then, he made the commitment to read the entire series on his own each summer and has done so four times.

One of Brady's favorite details in the book is the invisibility cloak that Harry's father handed down to him. When Harry places the cloak over his head, he can move about Hogwarts unnoticed. Brady wanted an invisibility cloak desperately, but it was the one Harry Potter accessory not sold in stores. We had every wand, Hogwarts costume, and sorting hat on the market, but no invisibility cloak.

The concept of invisibility is exciting in theory, and scientists are even working on ways to make it a reality using cameras, reflections and other high-tech gadgets. But invisibility in the case of neurological functioning is a reference to the inability of others to perceive that a condition exists which impacts how a child processes the world around them. There are very real differences in the way Brady is wired, but because others can't see those differences, it can cause unrealistic expectations for behavior, performance, and social interactions. This is why I founded KIND Families, for Kids with Invisible Neurological Differences.

Before we go further, please understand that when I talk about the invisible neurological differences in my son, I do so with sincere deference to parents whose children's challenges are more apparent and limiting. I can only imagine how it is exponentially more difficult to parent a child with these conditions, especially one which threatens the child's ability to live a long and full life. For all the struggles we have faced, I am grateful everyday for all the things Brady is able to do.

But the hidden nature of neurodiversity can cause others to react more harshly. The measure of grace that is naturally conditioned when interacting with someone who is visibly impacted evaporates and judgment sometimes takes its place.

I remember taking Brady on a plane to visit John's mom in Grand Junction, Colorado, when he was freshly diagnosed with autism. It was not the first time we had flown with him, so we were prepared for the trip. We had a book of *Wiggles* and *Curious George* DVDs and the portable DVD player, fully charged, in the backpack. We had lots of fruity squeeze treats to alleviate the ear pressure on takeoff, and we had his favorite stuffed animal by his side. We gave Brady the window seat, and he was elated to find he could see outside the plane.

He was fascinated by the takeoff and diminishing earth below, but once we hit 10,000 feet and unhooked his seatbelt Brady found a new passion—the window screen. He was hooked. It was like magic – he pulled down on the handle and the sky was gone, but when he pushed the screen up the sky was back! What fun!

He was having the time of his life. Up, down, up, down. Smiling and flapping his hands between each cycle. I hadn't even noticed that the screen was making a sound as it tapped the bottom and top of the window, I was just enjoying the pure joy on Brady's face as he played with his new toy.

Suddenly, an older woman in the middle seat in front of me whirled around and gave me a death glare through the gap in the backrests. "Will you make him STOP! For God's sake he's giving me a headache!" I was stunned. I never handle it well when someone yells at me, and while I fought to hold back tears, my stomach immediately went on spin cycle. The sound of Brady's activity wasn't even loud to me, in fact the rhythmic nature of it was almost lost behind the constant roar of the airplane engines.

Now I wasn't sure what to do. My people-pleaser instinct told me to pull Brady away from the window. If I encounter hostility from others, I usually go overboard attempting to diffuse the situation. But I also knew what would happen if I complied. I looked over at John for direction, and he shrugged his shoulders and nodded as if we should accept our fate.

I reached over and grabbed Brady under the arms and started to pull him to me. At first, he just bent his knees and resisted with a low whine, pulling away. He wriggled free of my grip and grabbed the handle to resume his fun. At that point the wicked witch of 23B decided I needed supervision to get the job done, so she turned around again and stared at me to make sure I finished the job. To her, I'm sure Brady looked like any other child, one who should take direction from his mother and obey her every command. But he wasn't like every other child.

Under her punishing gaze, I grabbed Brady again and pulled him into my lap, telling him in a high-pitched sing-song voice that we couldn't play with the window anymore. Mount Brady erupted. He leaned across his empty seat reaching desperately for the window screen, but I held him fast, sustaining the kicks and wails as he protested using every part of his body and every decibel of his voice. I tried to explain to him that he was bothering people with the window, which was almost laughable now that the whole plane was involved in his full-blown tantrum.

My new nemesis turned around to scowl at me again as I struggled to keep Brady contained. I looked her dead in the eye and snapped, "Is this better?" She turned around in a huff and all the souls on the plane dealt with the aftermath for the rest of the flight. When we arrived in Grand Junction an hour later, I'm sure the airport bar saw a spike in alcohol sales.

Invisibility was both a blessing and a curse in the early years of our autism journey. It helped us keep the truth about Brady's neurodiversity a secret in many situations. During short interactions in public with others, I could pretend to be a regular mom. It was my personal invisibility cloak, but it didn't always work. I was always waiting for the big reveal that would sneak up on us, the cloak falling to the ground and leaving others with a vision of a perfectly typical-looking child with his bad mother who couldn't manage him. Strangers didn't understand what was going on in his brain. Frankly, we didn't either. There were so many characteristics of autism we didn't grasp. We asked Brady how he felt, but for the first few years, his language delays kept him from answering.

When John and I decided to tell Brady about his autism and ADHD he was getting ready to start second grade at Lexis Preparatory, a school specifically for kids with learning disabilities. We were several years past our initial realization that Brady was on the spectrum, and any misconceptions we had about autism being a short-term problem were long gone.

I had also started to really lean into my faith, and part of that process involved a heart shift. Gradually our lies of omission about Brady's diagnosis became increasingly unsettling. Plus, once we started attending this particular school, the cat would be out of the proverbial bag. This was not a school for neurotypical children, so we finally started to reconsider our silence on the subject, both with outsiders, and with Brady himself.

The day after our big reveal to Brady about the way his brain works, I took him to get a haircut. Haircuts used to be a major ordeal, but over the years he thankfully made peace with a stranger coming at his head with a pair of sharp scissors. When the barber was finished with the trim she asked if he would like gel in his hair. To my shock and surprise Brady replied, "No, I don't like gel in my hair, because I have an autism brain."

You could have heard a pin drop in the salon for a split second, then everyone started giggling. There it was, we were out in the open, in a public place, and everyone in that store knew Brady was autistic. Brady owned it, and people were okay with it. It was time for us to own it too.

The last thing we wanted to do was convey to Brady that autism was something he should hide or be ashamed about. We encouraged him that he didn't need to make a formal announcement wherever he went like he did in the barbershop, but if he wanted to tell people he knew and trusted about how his brain works, he could. Autism is a part of him and always will be, like his curly brown hair.

John and I finally became more open about Brady's autism, especially since we attended a school where autism was just one of many diagnoses represented. Honesty was refreshing, empowering, and freeing. Being open with others also highlighted that sometimes I inadvertently let the invisibility of Brady's condition pull the wool over my own eyes. There are times I forget Brady has autism.

In some respects, my amnesia is a function of acceptance. More and more, I can let autism slip from the front of my mind to a quiet corner in the back. I can enjoy my son for his gifts, talents, and purpose. I can let the joy of Brady's heart be squarely at the center of my focus. In those times autism simply becomes a word, six letters in the dictionary without power or influence over our lives.

But other times I forget autism when I shouldn't. Especially during times of frustration. Like when I am trying to leave the house in a hurry and Brady is moving at sloth speed. Or when he loses the 432nd water bottle of the school year.

When Brady was younger, he couldn't tolerate hot food. I would cook his frozen chicken nuggets, and then put them back in the freezer for five minutes. The process was a delicate exercise to manage. Too long in the freezer and I'd have to microwave the chicken again. Too short, and he would scream and spit his food out in dramatic fashion. I would frequently buckle under the pressure and shout, "It's not hot! Just eat it already!"

Then one day Brady used his newfound grasp on language that age and lots of speech therapy gave him. He told me, "Mommy, what feels like room temperature to you feels burning hot to me." Boom. There it was. For the first time I had the slightest yet clearest understanding of what it felt like to be Brady. His invisible condition was real, and it impacted him in ways I was only beginning to grasp.

I fell into the same trap as a stranger on the street—wondering why this perfectly handsome healthy kid didn't just act...you know ...normal. It hurts to even write that. Especially since I know now that I wouldn't have him any other way.

A couple of weeks after Brady started his new school, the teacher met me at pickup and told me a story. The class was talking about anxiety, and what may cause a person to be anxious. Brady raised his hand and told the class that if someone didn't know they had autism and didn't understand why things were hard, it could make them anxious. That'll preach. Brady's condition isn't just invisible to strangers, it is sometimes invisible to us, and it was even invisible to him. When Brady looked in the mirror and saw a kid who looked just like his peers, he didn't understand why he struggled in areas of his life which came naturally to his classmates.

We all have parts of ourselves we don't want others to see. We try to pull the invisibility cloak over our insecurities, our imperfections, and our inadequacies, but the constant effort to hide who we really are just deepens our unease. We wait for the curtain to rise, revealing to the world that the great and powerful Oz we are pretending to be is just an ordinary old humbug.

Dropping the invisibility cloak may not always work the way we hope. Regretfully, it didn't work for Curtis's dad in the trampoline park that day. I did not show grace, and that short interaction forced me into years of silence about Brady's autism. Had I been honest about Brady's autism with the lady in 23B, would she have shown some grace and let him continue playing with the window screen? Maybe not. But we can't control others' actions and reactions, we can only choose how we respond.

Here's an idea. Instead of an invisibility cloak, what if we wore the armor of God? In Ephesians, Paul tells us God's version of outerwear will help us stand firm in truth and readiness. God will embolden us when we embrace the perfectly imperfect creations we are. Wearing God's cloak, no one can diminish our worth or damage our identity. Not even the lady in 23B.

CHAPTER 11
MRS. AVOCADO, THE HERO

Many years back I became an amateur connoisseur of avocado toast. I can't remember the first time I tried the dish, but I have always loved avocados on sandwiches, salads, or omelets, and I would almost always pay the extra $0.75 to add the smooth, buttery fruit to my meal. Avocado toast is fun to order because it's kind of like tiramisu —every chef or short order cook puts their own spin on it. Free tip—there is a place in northern Idaho called the Pack River General Store, and they have what I believe is the best avocado toast on the planet. They use inch-thick homemade bread as the base and top the mashed avocado with crema sauce, over easy eggs, and thick cut bacon. You need a steak knife to eat it! You're welcome.

John and I usually have the same five-ingredient protein shake for breakfast every day, but one morning I was out of almond milk, so we improvised. I had some ripe avocados in my fruit basket, and while I didn't have fresh bread either (it must have been that kind of week) I found some Eggos in the freezer. While the waffles were browning, I sliced the avocado carefully around the pit, spooned out the green delight and mashed it with a fork until it was chunky. I remembered the menu descriptions at some of my favorite restaurants, and after spreading the avocado generously on the toasted waffle, I added a light spray of extra virgin olive oil, "everything bagel" seasoning, sliced hard boiled eggs, and topped it with salt and pepper. Voila! It was delicious, and John loved it.

One time I served it for breakfast when John's aunt and uncle were visiting from rural New Jersey. They had never heard of avocado toast before, so it made me feel very sophisticated to serve them such a fancy treat. They were instant fans. Uncle Larry even took pictures of the plate with his phone and asked me for the recipe, a phenomenon that rarely happens with a product from my kitchen.

Brady was still little when my interest in the worldwide variations of avocado toast started to bloom. Like most kids on the autism spectrum, he was a VERY picky eater, and the visual appearance and texture of most foods made him reluctant to branch out. Especially if something on the plate was green.

Brady's approved menu selections fell in the orange-brown slice of the color wheel: goldfish crackers, chicken nuggets, and Beefaroni. He wouldn't touch other traditional "kid-friendly foods" like pizza, mac and cheese, hamburgers, or hot dogs. I can't explain how Beefaroni fit into Brady's aesthetic parameters, but I bought the cans in bulk. Of course, I was careful to pick the version with "no artificial preservatives" on the label, which in my flawed logic meant it was healthy, or at least non-toxic. I even got in the habit of traveling with cans of Beefaroni to make sure there would be something Brady would eat if nuggets weren't on the menu.

One time on a cub scout camping trip I packed a pop-top can of Beefaroni, knowing Brady wouldn't touch any of the fire smoked barbecue options. One mother, who was a particularly healthy eater, caught me as I opened the can and handed it to Brady with a plastic spoon. (Room temperature canned goods were also a perfect solution for Brady's aversion to hot foods. Two birds, one stone.)

As Brady dug in, the mom couldn't help herself and asked, "You're going to let him eat THAT??" I decided to turn my annoyance into sarcasm and replied. "Oh yes, it's awesome—I can feed him just like a cat. I don't even have to heat it up." She didn't hang out with us much for the rest of the trip.

When Brady was old enough to understand the value of money, we started to pay him a dollar for every new food he would try. However, many times the money just wasn't enough for him to take the risk of something yucky hitting his taste buds. With all of this in mind, I didn't consider that my avocado toast affinity had even reached his consciousness.

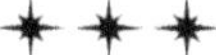

Brady's first grade teacher was a lovely woman who adored Brady. She had an adult daughter with some special needs, so she understood Brady's challenges and supported him with any accommodation he needed to be successful academically. The Friday before Mother's Day each year she hosted a brunch for all the first-grade moms. Parents of older kids who had been in her class raved about the event, so I should have been looking forward to it, but I wasn't.

Part of it was my nature—school parties usually involved some kind of craft, and I am not crafty. In fact, I tend to avoid anything that requires cutting, pasting, or gluing. I don't like the mess and I'm pretty sure the result will not be worth the effort. I attended a women's event at church around the same time, and the first activity was a craft. If I hadn't caught a ride to the event, I probably would have walked out.

The hosts explained that we were making picture frames and handed me some decorative supplies and a glue gun. I had never held a glue gun in my hand before, and fumbled as I tried to load it, burning myself and dripping hot glue on the white tablecloth in the process. One of the organizers sweetly gave me some instructions and safety tips, but couldn't conceal her wonder that a woman in her forties had somehow missed out on learning such a critical life skill.

Crafts were not the main reason I was anxious for the Mother's Day party, however. Brady really struggled behaviorally during class celebrations. His routine was blown to bits, the small room was loud and chaotic, and he was not interested in participating in forced group games with the other kids. When Brady was overwhelmed, his response was to run, so at most parties I spent my time chasing after him, dragging him back to the room and begging him to participate. All the while, I painted a smile on my sweaty face and pretended I was enjoying myself like all the other moms. But I knew my illusion was flimsy at best, and completely transparent at worst.

The other families knew something was different about Brady, mostly due to the full-time aide who helped him in the classroom until the end of kindergarten. Some parents were curious and asked politely why he needed an aide, and I answered with the same scripted response—he just has some developmental delays. Other, less compassionate moms seemed to make Brady the topic of the school parking lot conversation before pickup. I couldn't be sure they were talking about us, but the expressions on their faces and the frequent glances my way supported my suspicions.

I never mentioned autism with anyone other than teachers at the school. I was afraid if other parents were as ignorant about autism as I was a few years earlier, Brady could be ostracized, bullied, or worse. But eventually the gossip gang couldn't resist, and I was outed in front of the whole class while volunteering for Pioneer Day, just a few months before Mother's Day.

She approached me in a whirlwind, so I had no time to prepare.

"Oh my gosh! So, I heard Brady has autism! He doesn't look autistic." The skinny, tall blonde smiled and looked at me like she just commented on my purse, not my son. I wanted to ask what she thought autism looked like, but I couldn't speak. I searched my brain for a pithy comeback, but none materialized. The other moms became instantly silent as she went on, "So I heard Jenny McCarthy had a son with autism, but she cured him so that's good news, right?!" I stammered out a weak excuse and walked away, my heart pounding in my chest.

I am sure it took about a nanosecond for the moms within earshot to spread the news that Brady was autistic. The grapevine at the school was like a bullet train. I could feel the stares in the parking lot intensify, and some moms were distant and nervous around me.

Regardless, I didn't want to miss the Mother's Day breakfast. At this point we already knew we were leaving the school, and I didn't want to let Brady or his teacher down, so I convinced myself I could make it through one last day.

The morning of the party I quickly understood why this event had earned all the accolades—this was no Dunkin' Donut social. The moms lined up outside the door and waited to be let in. When the door opened, we walked in single file. I noticed classical music playing softly in the background, and I smelled the sweet scent of fancy candles burning on the teacher's desk. All the kids' desks had been grouped together and covered in linen tablecloths, and each grouping had a vase of fresh flowers in the center.

Finally, I saw Brady, and he grabbed my hand and led me to my seat. "Mrs. Baker" was written in calligraphy on a canvas name card which was propped up by a costume tiara he instructed me to wear. In front of me was a fancy paper plate and doily with two delectable pastries, a cup of mixed fruit, and a mandarin orange. Next to the plate was a gift wrapped in red, black and white polka dot paper—the teacher's signature style. After a quick prayer, the kids sat down on the carpet and it was time to eat. Brady was being a model child. They must have practiced this, I thought.

After breakfast we opened our presents—homemade scrapbooks with pictures of the kids taken during the year, notes about the things they loved about Mom, and even a page that had a pocket with "coupons" we could redeem for various chores or shows of affection. The book was decorated with ribbons and embellished paper and to this day is one of my most favorite gifts from Brady. I had to admit, so far this party was going great. Brady was calm and following the example of the other kids, and I was able to eat and chat in peace.

Once all the plates and cups had been cleared (by the kids no less) it was time for the big surprise—each student had written a story called "My Mom, The Superhero." One by one, each child walked up to the podium and read about their mom's superpower. The superpowers for each mom were pretty similar—kindness, love, kisses, hugs, characteristics that would make a mom melt, and by the tears in the room, each kid hit the mark.

When it was Brady's turn I couldn't wait to hear about all the attributes that Brady thought were super about me. He walked to the front with his stapled pink report and started to read confidently.

"My mom is a real superhero. You might think her name is Kari, but it is really Mrs. Avocado."

Wait, what? My mind tried to process what I just heard, but it was difficult to think because the entire room erupted in laughter. The teacher put her hand on his shoulder to have him wait for the audience to quiet down, and when they did, she motioned for him to continue.

"My Mom's superpower is making the best avocado breakfast EVER!" More laughter. This was not going as I planned. Other moms got sweetness, hugs, and love, and I got avocado toast?? I longed at that moment to just be like everyone else. To just fit in. Just this once. But he went on and it was clear that was not going to happen today.

"One day my Mommy was at home with me and Auntie Kimberly. There was a big problem on the TV. There was a man saying that all the restaurants had run out of avocado breakfasts. People were very sad because they all wanted one."

I looked around and noticed the comments and giggles had died down. This was a story. Everyone appeared to listen as he continued.

"My Mom heard of this and saved the day. She went to the people. When she got there, she pushed a button on her superhero helmet and avocado breakfast flew out and was delivered to all of the people."

The visual hit home. Everyone in the room was smiling wider by the minute, and every eye was firmly planted on my son. He held his audience in rapt attention and my countenance started to soften. He concluded the story, "They cheered, as Mrs. Avocado disappeared in a cloud of avocado juice. I am so proud of my Mommy."

The classroom erupted in applause, as well as some whoops and hollers. Brady lowered his paper and bowed dramatically with the final word, "The End."

I sat stunned, processing the scene in the room and the message in Brady's story. I'm not sure what avocado juice is, but at least Mrs. Avocado went out with a bang. The other moms were genuinely impressed, and some, I daresay, were jealous. All the letters from the other children sounded the same, but I got to be Mrs. Avocado! In that moment no one saw autism. Everyone saw Brady. They saw his creativity, his heart, and his gifts on display.

I will admit, initially I was disappointed when I thought Brady had bypassed the chance to compliment me on all my wonderful motherly qualities, especially in front of women I thought were questioning my aptitude for motherhood. But my expectation that he would read a flowery poem of traditional love and devotion was misplaced. That's not Brady.

You see, emotions are difficult for kids with autism. Feelings are hard to control, and even harder to express. Brady recognized my love for avocado toast, and used his flair for storytelling to show me what he thinks of me: I help people who are sad and save the day. Best of all, he is proud of me. This was so much better than any cookie-cutter praise he could have copied and pasted from a template. Now as Brady came over to hug me, I couldn't stop the tears.

Maybe you have been there, wishing you could fit in, or that your experience could be like everyone else's. I get it. I wanted desperately to be like the other moms in Brady's class, to be ordinary. But those moms didn't get to become the hearty green superhero of their kid's imagination. Our paths are all different by design, and we can get so wrapped up hoping for ordinary, we might not see the extraordinary right in front of us.

Remember, God created each one of us with specific skills, talents, and personality traits that are designed to have an impact on the world. We all have weaknesses to bear, and abilities to share. While social skills and team sports don't come naturally to Brady, writing, drawing, and reading are second nature. Stop comparing and start celebrating what makes you unique. Many times, our differences are really our superpowers in disguise.

CHAPTER 12 DRAWiNG PiCTURES

Transitions are hard for everyone, regardless of how our brains are wired. There is something about the familiar that acts like an anchor to our psyche—even if the familiar isn't all that great. Maybe you have been stuck in a job that didn't fulfill you, but you didn't leave because it paid the bills. Or you've been in a relationship that wasn't healthy, but you stayed because you thought it was better than being alone. Maybe you have had the same ugly picture from your husband's bachelor pad hanging on your living room wall for twelve years but it's still there because you don't have the time, energy, or design expertise to replace it (sorry, that one might just be me). Then you get it. Transitions can be scary, exhausting, and disruptive, and sometimes we avoid them even if it provides the promise of something better. As author Isaac Asimov wrote, "Life is pleasant. Death is peaceful. It's the transition that's troublesome."

Transitions are especially tough for kids with autism and other neurological differences. And it's not just the big transitions like moving or changing schools that are the problem. For Brady it was often transitions that seem routine to you and me that caused the most tears: leaving the house to get into the car, putting down a toy to do homework, or turning off the TV to go to bed. Ripping Brady away from an activity without warning, especially a preferred one, could be a recipe for disaster when he was younger.

One afternoon when Brady was five I picked him up from a visit at my parents' house to take him to his weekly occupational therapy appointment. Another autism mom I talked to right after we realized Brady may have autism had suggested we start OT right away. Don't wait for the diagnosis, she warned. Just do it. I didn't even know what OT was at the time, but at that point I would have signed him up for kazoo classes if someone told me to. It was the right move as Brady's evaluation revealed he was severely delayed with his gross and fine motor skills; the exact functions OT would address.

Miss Lisa was his first therapist, and Brady connected with her quickly. She was warm and kind, but firm, and she made therapy fun for Brady with games, toys, and motion tools like roller boards and balance beams. Since this was my first experience with OT, I was pleasantly surprised that he wasn't going to be strapped to a torture chair for an hour each week. The exercises were all play-based, and while he struggled with some activities which tested the boundaries of his fine and gross motor abilities, he relished the individual attention she gave him, and never complained about his sessions in almost two years.

That was about to change. Brady and I usually drove to OT straight from school, but today was a holiday, and my parents had been watching him so I could take a work call in peace. I picked him up from their house with no issues, and we headed to the hospital. We arrived about ten minutes later and got out of the car in front of the sliding glass doors, and warmly greeted the hospital valets we had come to know by name. I reached into the passenger seat and grabbed his oversized activity bag, my purse, and water bottles, then hopped down and opened the back door to unlock the strap on his car seat and lift him to the ground. I took his hand in mine and we walked absentmindedly through the doors into the lobby.

Suddenly, as we stepped onto the shiny tile floor, he snatched his hand out of mine, threw himself to the ground on his hands and knees and started crying, "No, no, no, no!" What felt like dozens of people stopped what they were doing to look disapprovingly at my son's public display, surely thinking I was the most terrible mother in the world.

I knelt down and spoke softly to him that we needed to get up and get on the elevator, feeling the stares of the gaping audience around us. But my voice did not calm Brady—instead it caused him to flip over onto his back, kicking and writhing as his screams of protest intensified. I didn't know what else to do except to pick him up—all 50 pounds of him—along with my bags, bottles, and other accessories. Needless to say, at the moment I needed three more arms than the good Lord gave me as I tried to wrestle him off the ground. I dropped my water bottle and some sweet soul came over and asked if she could help, but I declined her assistance, grabbed the bottle and kept my focus on forward progress toward the elevator. I was sweating and my face was hot, but after what seemed like the battle of the century we crossed the threshold of the elevator and the doors closed behind us. Finally in the privacy and safety of the elevator I was able to put him down, but when we reached the fourth floor, I had to drag him to the clinic door by the arm like I was leading an animal to slaughter.

The therapist must have heard the commotion (or possibly someone called her from downstairs), and before we reached the door she walked out, took a hold of Brady's hand and told me to go downstairs and get some coffee. I was confused. I had never left him in therapy before—I didn't know that was even an option. I assumed she would want an explanation of our intense arrival. But she looked at me with understanding eyes and told me she could handle it, opened the door, and she and Brady disappeared behind it.

I stood there for a few moments, almost unable to move. I noticed an exit sign above the door next to me and almost fell through the door. I collapsed onto the cold cement stairs and cried so hard my stomach started to cramp. Once I caught my breath my mind started racing. What could have caused this? I tried to piece together the day and immediately thought of my parents. That was it! It had to be. They must have given him some sugary toxic treat with number 5 yellow dye and possibly crack cocaine that caused this meltdown. They had been known to take grandparent privileges when it came to unhealthy snacks.

I called them on my phone and through tears practically accused them of poisoning my son. They were devastated while they tried to explain that the only food they gave him was goldfish, a pre-approved and Mom-sanctioned snack. No, this was not about food. Something sparked a reaction in my son's brain that was so primal that his fight or flight instinct took over his entire body. I finally calmed down enough to explain and apologize to my parents, and God bless them by the time we hung up the phone they were on their way to the hospital. They were afraid I would need help getting him home, and this time, I didn't decline the help.

I went downstairs and ordered a hot tea, and my parents showed up about fifteen minutes later. We talked through the episode briefly but mostly just sat in silence waiting to go back upstairs. When his session was almost over we returned to the fourth floor and I walked slowly to the door, not sure what to expect and not sure if I had the strength to deal with whatever awaited me. I walked in and found Brady playing on the floor with his therapist showing no signs of the events less than an hour earlier.

For the longest time I didn't understand what sparked the outburst that day, but looking back now, I believe it was related to transitions. I picked Brady up from a preferred activity, and took him to a less preferred activity without warning, and the result was explosive.

Most of the time Brady's meltdowns were not as dramatic as the hospital incident, but we struggled regularly with transitions and were grateful when we learned some tricks of the trade in one of the parent training sessions we attended. Interestingly, we learned the key to transitions is to transition the transition. That is not a typo. It just means that you must provide a gentler slide from one activity to the next, rather than pulling the child abruptly out of what they are presently engaged in.

After some practice we got pretty good at the pre-transition countdown. For instance, before leaving the house we would give several warnings it was nearing go-time. Ten minutes before we would give Brady the first notification that we would need to get in the car soon. Then we would give a five-minute warning, then a one-minute warning. The key was to limit the surprise factor and set the expectation for what was coming next. However, that did not provide Brady with a roadmap for the whole day, only for the next event. If the next activity was a less desirable one, the countdowns were not as effective. We needed something more, and it dawned on us that we already had a model to draw from.

At the beginning of every OT session, Miss Lisa would draw out a list of exercises Brady needed to complete that day to get to his reward, which was usually a few minutes in the large platform swing that hung from the ceiling in the corner. Brady had some input into the order of the chores, and sometimes even the authority to pick one thing over another. She would draw the schedule of how they would spend their hour, and as they completed each step, Brady could cross it off the list.

It worked, because each time he crossed off a non-preferred task, I could see him celebrate a little. He knew each step meant he was getting closer to finishing his work and collecting his reward. Brady responded well to this strategy and very rarely had a problem getting everything accomplished in OT. I am the same way, and maybe you are too. I work better from a list. If I have too much to do I can't remember it all without writing it down, and I also love crossing things off my list! Brady wasn't reading fluently yet, so I needed to provide him with visual interpretations of the transitions he could expect during the whole day—start to finish.

So, I decided to give it a try, and after a few days we had a routine. Each morning I would take a simple piece of white copy paper attached to a clipboard and draw perpendicular lines to make boxes for each step of our day. Brady would sit at the counter next to me watching, as I would fill in each square with crude and quick drawings of the events that would lead us from breakfast to bedtime that day.

Here is Brady eating breakfast. Then we will get dressed and brush our teeth. Then we will get into the car. Then we will go into school. Then we will get back in the car. Then we will go to Miss Lisa's for OT. Then, then, then. You get the picture. Pun intended.

I am not gifted with any artistic ability, but I got pretty good at drawing an outline of my small SUV and stick figures of the important people who were part of our daily routine. My sister had long curly hair and glasses, my mom, short hair, I had shoulder length hair flipped at the end. Everyone including teachers and therapists had their own minimalistic doppelganger, good enough for Brady to recognize.

Every morning Brady got a sneak peak of the future—a daily still-frame movie of what was to come. The process was monotonous, but effective. I knew I could purchase picture cards to take the place of the repetitive drawings, or even make copies, but the process of creating the pictures seemed as important to Brady as seeing the final result. Watching me draw each box allowed him to digest the information piece by piece, versus having to understand the full picture all at once. It also gave him some input in the process—he got to ask questions along the way, and even corrected me if I forgot a step. If I left out one of our driving boxes he would ask, "Mommy, how are we getting home from school?"

Transitions became easier with Brady after we started our new morning ritual. It wasn't perfect, as unexpected surprises would pop up occasionally, but we could always draw ourselves back to some point on the schedule that he had planned for that morning. If nothing else, we could make it to bedtime.

I understand why Brady found comfort in the picture process. Providing structure to his expectations allowed him time to prepare for each transition in advance and mitigate the fight or flight response. If Brady had known that fateful morning that we were going to leave my parents' house and go directly to OT, maybe he wouldn't have reacted so strongly once we got there.

We all react differently to transitions in our life. Since the only constant in life is change, we can't avoid them, but still, they can be unsettling. Especially if you are a planner like me. Unexpected transitions can cause anxiety, fear, and foreboding. A diagnosis like autism forces you to transition from the life you pictured to a new reality. For me, I had to shift from a working wife and mother to a full-time CEO of my child's development.

Even transitions you know are coming require you to relinquish your misguided perception of control. Think about having a baby. You have months to prepare your heart and mind for the transition from carefree couple to parents, but the only way to truly understand how different your life will be is to walk through it. God is the illustrator of our days. Sometimes I wish He would show us the entire book up front, but instead he gives us just enough light to walk with Him to the next page. We have to trust Him to be our guide.

Eventually Brady learned to read proficiently, and I was able to use words instead of pictures to lay the groundwork for his day. Now that he is in middle school his schedule is more general and only varies by after-school appointments or sports, so instead of a daily detailed visual we use a dry erase calendar with days of the week. We still make paper lists when he has a heavy homework load to complete or lots of chores to finish, otherwise we save the paper and update the dry erase board each Sunday. I'm sure the trees are as grateful as I am.

CHAPTER 13
BEES AND SQUiRRELS

Like many kids with autism and ADHD, Brady has a tendency to hyperfocus on preferred subjects or thoughts. Once a topic or idea makes it to the top of the Brady brain chart, distracting him with anything else is a feat. His first extreme interest was *The Wiggles* and specifically the DVD covers, but over the years his interests shifted to Winnie the Pooh, then space shuttle launches, Superman and Batman, capuchin monkeys, and finally to *Star Wars.*

Star Wars stuck, and it stuck like superglue. You have no idea the details and obscure trivia this kid has retained and can regurgitate on demand. He has watched every original, prequel, and sequel, every series, cartoon, and YouTube video relating to *Star Wars* known to man, and he somehow has the ability to reconcile each one's time and placement in the grand scheme of the canon. I used to consider myself a *Star Wars* fan, but on the relative spectrum of fandom, I am teetering on the precipice of one side and Brady is not even in my line of sight on the other.

John and I are just thankful the focus of his attention is no longer *The Wiggles.* For the rest of my life, I won't be able to see fruit salad without "yummy, yummy" going through my head. True *Wiggles* fans will understand.

Hyperfocus can be a superpower if used in a healthy way. Many of the world's greatest creative minds like Elon Musk and Steve Jobs have brains that are wired similarly to Brady's, and their ability to be unwavering in their attention is a factor of their success. I've often wished that my brain had a super focus setting because even if I love the activity, it won't take long for me to drift into another lane.

Unfortunately, sometimes our greatest strengths also highlight our greatest weakness. While Brady has no problem focusing on things he loves for hours on end, sometimes he becomes so immersed he completely blocks out the world. We call it "Rock Brain."

Rock Brain is one of the "Unthinkables," who are fictional cartoon villains created by Michelle Garcia Winner to help kids visualize behavior problems that keep them from socially acceptable interactions with others. Rock Brain makes people get stuck on their ideas and can only be combated with Rex Flexinator, who helps you be a flexible thinker so you don't get stuck. I always pictured Rex with an Arnold Schwarzenegger-esque accent.

When Rock Brain attacked Brady, it was very difficult to transition Brady away from a topic or activity. But in its worst representation, Rock Brain would use his evil powers to push Brady into what we called "sad moments."

From the time he was able to talk, Brady would have sudden, unexplained changes in his mood. We would be on the couch watching *The Wiggles* and he would go from singing and dancing to crying in what seemed like an instant. We tried to figure out what caused the dramatic swings, but he didn't have the language skills to explain his feelings to us.

Once a sad moment started, there was little John or I could say or do to pull Brady back to us. When Brady was very young and unable to communicate, he would bang his head on the counter or wall. As he got older and had more words available, he would tell us he needed to be punished and would suggest options that were often draconian and severe. Usually, he would pick out something we knew he loved like a stuffed animal, and ask us to throw it away, take it to the dump, or burn it. Or he would say he didn't want to see our family anymore, that we weren't good for him anymore, that he didn't love us anymore.

We would beg him to understand that he wasn't in trouble, and we had no reason to punish him, but nothing worked. It was like a thief snuck in my house and stole my happy sweet boy and replaced him with a look-a-like shell. During these spells, his brain seemed to be on a constant loop that was stuck on the negative, like Eeyore invaded his soul. Most of the time we had no idea what triggered the episode, but the only cure seemed to be time. The therapists told us we were feeding the behavior by pleading with him to stop, so they wanted us to let him have quiet time in his room, alone. Eventually he would emerge, and it would be as if the episode never happened. Like a prolonged hit-and-run accident with the perpetrator, Rock Brain, escaping without a trace.

When Brady was getting ready to enter kindergarten, we drove to California for a quick summer escape. Brady was in his car seat in the back, watching *The Bee Movie* for the first time on the small portable DVD player. I was excited that he was trying a new show. Up until that time he had a small selection of DVDs he would watch, and I knew each of the scripts by heart. From my vantage point in the front seat, Brady was loving the film, giggling, and clapping along. I remember being thankful for peace in the car.

Of course, Murphy's Law kicked in and suddenly Brady started to cry. He screamed for us to stop the movie, so I frantically unbuckled my seatbelt, whirled around to face him, grabbed the player and fumbled with the stop button. I was too late. The damage was done. The sad moment took over and he became a bundle of tears and despair.

We asked him what happened, but he couldn't explain. I played the video in my lap to make sure it hadn't skipped or gotten stuck, but it was running fine, and there were no surprise horror movie scenes spliced into the cartoon that would have caused such a reaction. He was so distraught we considered turning around and canceling the trip, but we didn't. We dealt with the aftermath of the Rock Brain attack from Yuma to San Diego.

When I was in the corporate world I attended lots of conferences and heard lots of keynote speakers. It didn't matter what the overarching message was—getting more clients, being more present with your family, being a better manager—the suggestion always included a discussion of "mindset." If you want to sell more, you must have the right mindset. If you want to achieve a goal, you must have the right mindset. If you want to be a better wife, mother, friend, you name it, you must have the right mindset.

We need a growth mindset, a service mindset, an abundance mindset. Anyone else getting exhausted thinking about mindset? I'm not saying the advice isn't helpful, and I don't deny the scientific research that says we can change the neural pathways of our brains to create different outcomes in our lives. But when Brady got sad, I couldn't tell him to change his mindset.

I needed a tool to snap the thread of thoughts circling his brain when the sadness overtook him. Time alone eventually helped, but we didn't know if it would take ten minutes or two hours. We tried everything else, including *Star Wars*-themed motivators, to bring him back to us, but he was in a galaxy far, far away and not even Luke Skywalker could help.

Then one Sunday our church had a guest speaker, Dr. Lori Maldonado, who gave me an idea. She was talking about how the Bible provides strategies for dealing with anxiety, and while I'd never thought of Brady's episodes as reflections of anxiety, I started to consider the possibility. She reminded us that the Bible prescribes a very specific treatment for anxiety, which is found in the book of Philippians.

You see, Paul wrote the book of Philippians while he was in prison, yet it is considered one of the most joy-filled books of the Bible. If anyone had a right to complain, it was Paul, however he declared in chapter 4 that we are to "Rejoice in the Lord always." He didn't say, "Rejoice in the Lord only when things are going your way." He said always, and he meant always.

Paul continued by telling us not to worry about anything. I know, that doesn't sound possible, especially if you are dealing with trials in your life such as a child with special needs. But his instruction wasn't just an empty directive; he told us what to do instead of worrying. Pray. About everything. Be thankful for what we have, and pray. And God will bring you peace. He didn't say God will fix everything. He said you will have peace.

But beyond praying, you must focus your mind on something other than the circumstance that is causing you anxiety. That is the hard part for all of us, right? When trouble appears, the issue can quickly consume our thoughts. Whether we are trying to solve the problem or wallow in its misery, we have a hard time getting it out of our head unless we have something else to take its place.

Remember *Raiders of the Lost Ark*? When the movie starts, Indiana Jones wants to take a valuable artifact from its resting place, but he knows he has to replace it with something the same weight or else the booby traps will be activated. He fills a bag with sand and very carefully, very quickly, takes the item off its perch and slides the sandbag in its place. For a moment he thinks he's home free, but then he winds up getting chased by natives with spears and a large rolling ball. Why? Because there wasn't enough sand in the bag to match the weight of the artifact.

When we try to replace negative thoughts in our life, the new thought must have as much or more weight, or power, than the negative thought, or else the new thought will sink under the weight of your negativity. For most of us, we can't overcome anxiety and crushing despair by thinking of pumpkin spice lattes. Although, that may work for my sister. You need an arsenal of goodness that is ready for you to draw upon.

Thankfully Paul gave us a framework to find just the right arrows to fill our quiver. In Philippians 4:8 he wrote, "Whatever is true, whatever is honorable, whatever is just, whatever is pure, whatever is lovely, whatever is commendable—if there is any moral excellence and if there is anything praiseworthy—dwell on these things."

There's your mindset. It's a fill in the blank template that results in a personalized battle plan for anxiety and sadness. You can dwell on the hard things, or you can dwell on the things in your life that fit each one of those categories.

I decided to give Paul's advice a try with Brady. I found a verse card image on the internet, copied it to Word, and below it I created a space for Brady to tell me the things in his life that each powerful word described. For instance, Brady thought brownies were excellent, he thought capuchin monkeys were lovely, and our family was true. The best part is there are no wrong answers to this quiz.

TRUE = ______________________________
NOBLE = ______________________________
RIGHT = ______________________________
PURE = ______________________________
LOVELY = ______________________________
ADMIRABLE = ______________________________
EXCELLENT = ______________________________
PRAISEWORTHY = ______________________________

Once we got Brady's answers typed in, we laminated the list and posted it on a bulletin board in his room. When we would see a sad moment start to take its grip, we would direct Brady to the board, and ask him to think as hard as he could about everything on the list. I can't say it worked every time, but I do believe it helped to shorten the duration of the occurrences. A couple of times, as he got older and his interests changed, we reprinted the sheet with his current answers. Brownies became Baby Yoda.

Here's the thing. Even as adults we can't avoid sadness and turmoil on this side of heaven. We can usually pinpoint the cause, but not always. Philippians 4:8 provides us with a powerful weapon we can use to fight the sadness that will inevitably attack us in this broken world. It's a tool straight from God, so I trust it.

Fill out the list. Print it out and tape it to your computer monitor. Keep it in your wallet. And remember, the verse says to *dwell* on those things. Dwell doesn't mean let them flitter around in your brain along with thousands of squirrels and shiny things. It means *live* in them. Let them inhabit your mind, take up residence there, and overpower the darkness.

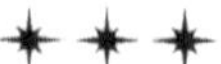

About a year ago, we saw an ad for *The Bee Movie* on television. We told Brady about what had happened in the car on that fateful trip to California and asked what set him off. He couldn't remember the incident, but we were all intrigued to see if we could figure it out, so we decided to watch it as a family.

The first part of the movie was cute, although a little strange. As someone who had an allergic reaction to yellowjacket stings as a child, the idea of a human forming a romantic relationship with a bee was a little hard to embrace. But we all laughed at the funny parts, and found nothing objectionable, until Winnie the Pooh appeared in a cameo.

The bees were taking back all the honey for themselves, and Winnie was on their most wanted list. A character resembling an FBI agent held a gun with its crosshairs on Pooh Bear's heart. The bee yelled, "Take him out!" Pooh was hit with a tranquilizer gun and fell off the log. Immediately after the shot the agent said Pooh would be fine in a couple of hours, but Brady didn't hear that the first time. In Brady's mind, Winnie the Pooh was dead. Shot mercilessly over a jar of honey. Pooh was one of Brady's most beloved stuffed animals, and the star of some of his favorite animated movies, and he had been killed in cold blood. At least in Brady's mind. That was the impetus of the hours-long sad moment that spanned two states.

We stopped the movie and stared incredulously at each other. We finally had answers to why Brady got stuck in his sadness that day, and frankly, I couldn't blame him. It was traumatizing. We all laughed at the revelation, especially Brady, who joked that he wanted to sue Jerry Seinfeld, the movie's producer, for infliction of pain and suffering.

It was exceedingly satisfying to finally understand the cause of one of Brady's sad moments. That bee got in Brady's bonnet, and it stuck. There were dozens more episodes over the years for which the origins would remain a mystery, but now we had a secret weapon. When a sad moment came, we would Philippians 4:8-it.

This is not just a tool for kids. Whether it's an illness, a broken relationship, or a child with special needs, we sometimes need to take our eyes off the elephant in the room and concentrate on the blessings all around it. Name the noble, name the true, name the excellent and praiseworthy. And when darkness and sadness fill your mind, make a choice about how you will respond. Either dwell *in* the hard, or dwell *on* the good.

CHAPTER 14
THE SOCiAL DiLEMMA

I was a huge fan of the TV show *Friends* in my twenties. Okay, I am still a huge fan. I frequently waste time that could surely be spent in more productive ways watching clips of the show from various Instagram pages. It has permanently changed the images that pop in my head when I hear the words "lobster" or "pivot." The acting and humor were flawless, but it was the relationships between the characters that made the show so powerful. They loved each other and they grew up together. I have been fortunate to have friends like that throughout most of the defining seasons of my life.

I have a tight group of sorority sisters from college who are like family. I have a beautiful band of God-loving women from church who walk with me in my faith. I have a fabulous foursome of fun fearless gals who were my constant companions as I entered and exited my forties. My bestie from that group even became pregnant right after I did so we could go through motherhood together. Way to take one for the team, Lisa! And of course, I now have my KIND mom tribe.

I just assumed it would be the same for Brady, and that making friends would come easily to him. Once again, autism had other plans.

Until recently, friends were not a priority for Brady. Difficulty with peer interaction is one of the signature challenges by which autism is characterized. Except for my friend Lisa's daughters who are more like family than friends, Brady spent much of his short life as a lone ranger. Ironically, he has always been great with adults, and thrives on their attention. His large vocabulary and tendency to speak like a sixty-year-old professor is endearing and novel to grownups but was often a barrier to building relationships with kids his own age.

For several years after the diagnosis, Brady had little interest in other kids. John and I would attend birthday parties with him and try to facilitate communication with other partygoers, but it was like trying to get the same pole of two magnets to connect. Like there was an invisible barrier between them. On a good day Brady would completely avoid and ignore the other kids, and on a bad day he would try to escape out into the street or have a meltdown.

It hit me hard that Brady wasn't bonding with other children, or even showing an interest in making friends. How did this social butterfly mama produce a child who would rather stay in a cocoon? If you have children, I'm betting they have some characteristics that make you wonder if the nurses played a little shell game with the babies at the hospital. Maybe your son has a high metabolism that allows him to eat like Jabba the Hutt and still fit into skinny jeans, while you eat a cookie and have to spend three hours at the gym to work it off. Or maybe you are a bookworm, and your kid hates reading. Or you are a sports fanatic, and your kid just wants to watch other people play video games on YouTube. Who knew that was a thing?

It's almost as if God purposefully gives us kids with contrasting qualities to give us some perspective. To help us understand that our view of the universe is distorted by our own experiences. How much more grace do we give to others when we realize the little person we are raising can have such a divergent outlook on life from our own. Maybe God thinks by teaching us to love our children's uniqueness, it will help us love others better too.

I prayed Brady would make friends with a neurotypical child at his first school, but it wasn't happening naturally. Most of his classmates were nice to him, but they knew he was different. He had a full-time aide in the classroom with him through kindergarten. In first grade he was independent, but he had visible support systems in place and therapists would visit the class regularly to observe. That dynamic caused there to be distance between Brady and the other children. To most of the kids, Brady was not like them. His behavior was a little out of the ordinary, he couldn't make eye contact, and his communication was impacted by his brain's processing speed and inability to "read the room."

Reading the room is a critical social skill that comes naturally to most of us, but for many kids on the spectrum reading social cues and facial expressions is like understanding a foreign language. Someone with deficits in this area may not recognize that someone is getting frustrated with him, or wants to change the subject, or wants to be left alone. For most people, that type of awareness is embedded in our consciousness.

For example, if you walk on a plane and sit down next to someone with AirPods in their ears and their eyes closed, do you try to start a conversation or let them be? I know there are some of you extreme extroverts who would jump in with an ice breaker question anyway, but most of us would read the cues, and leave our seatmate alone. Not Brady.

The summer before first grade we were swimming in a community pool, when Brady saw a kid a little older than him diving for little torpedo toys. The pool was not crowded, so there would have been plenty of room for the boys to play separately without incident, but we hadn't brought any pool toys, and Brady loved to dive for treasure. The first time the kid threw the toy, Brady blasted off toward the torpedo and snatched it from the bottom of the pool. The boy was not amused, retrieved the torpedo and told Brady very plainly, "Leave me alone." I swam over and tried to encourage Brady to head to the other side of the pool with me, but as soon as the torpedo started flying through the air, Brady was off again trying to snag it.

This time, the boy was not as even-tempered. He screamed, "I told you to leave me alone!" The outburst was paired with a death stare that could have scared Charles Manson, but Brady was oblivious. I scrambled to Brady and started pulling him away when another woman interjected from the side of the pool.

"Justin, who are you yelling at?" So much for my stealth escape. I went into fixer mode. I explained it was my son and apologized to her for the intrusion. I explained that Brady had developmental delays (you know, my secret code for autism) and that he didn't understand her son didn't want to play.

God bless that woman, she let Justin have it. The boy's death stare turned immediately to a scowl and eye roll. This time she apologized to me, and made Justin apologize to Brady. But deep down, I knew it was Brady who caused the problem, even if Justin's response was harsh. Justin made himself very clear he didn't want Brady to play with him, but Brady couldn't read the signs.

Most of us experience extreme embarrassment when we suddenly realize that our understanding of a situation doesn't match reality. Like the time my dad showed up at an Octoberfest work party in Lederhosen and was the only one in costume. Brady on the other hand, was not impacted by other peoples' reaction to his behaviors, so learning from his missteps was even harder. In some ways, it was a blessing that he wasn't hurt emotionally, but sometimes natural feedback is the best teacher.

I was concerned that Brady's social delays would only continue to get worse. Relating to peers becomes more and more nuanced with age. Think back to high school if you dare. It was a social minefield, and if you didn't step carefully, you could get blown up.

One of the staples in our therapy pantry from the time Brady was diagnosed with autism was social skills groups. Speech and language pathologists would pull together small groups of kids with similar levels of language function and hold supervised playdates to start conditioning the children to recognize and respond to social cues. The lessons started with role-play exercises to help teach how to read facial expressions. For instance, a girl would cross her arms, furrow her brow, and frown so the kids would deduce she was mad. Or a boy would pretend to cry demonstratively to show he was sad.

They graduated into discussing how our behaviors impact people's thoughts about us. If we act in an unexpected way, for instance with a sudden outburst or making strange noises, it could cause others to have different thoughts about us. The way someone thinks about us impacts the way they treat us. The leaders talked about emotional regulation, flexibility in play, taking turns, all things that Brady struggled with when he was in the presence of his peers. Most of the curriculum was based on Michele Garcia-Winner's books on social communication, the same author that brought us the dastardly Rock Brain.

During the summer, the organization that sponsored the social skills group put on a camp called "Kamp-Talk-A-Lot," and Brady attended every year. At the time, Brady tended to fill any semblance of silence with a conversation about one of his extreme interests, so John wondered if we could find a "Camp-Talk-Not-So-Much." But all kidding aside, the strategy was starting to work. The camps and groups allowed Brady to learn skills that didn't come naturally to him. I was just concerned that book smarts in this area wouldn't convert to street smarts.

There was one boy Brady met at Kamp-Talk-A-Lot who was also in his kindergarten class. From day one, Cody and Brady gravitated toward each other like magnets (this time, with opposite ends attracting). While Brady struggled to build relationships with neurotypical peers, he always seemed more comfortable with kids on the spectrum. It is as if Brady has some kind of autism radar.

Brady and Cody "parallel played" at first, meaning each did his own thing in proximity to each other. I was grateful he had at least one child with whom he could occupy a room and not try to escape. That is not to say that playdates were easy with two young boys on the spectrum. Often each boy's different obsessive interests and inflexibility resulted in tears and tantrums. Even so, as the boys spent more and more time together, their bond turned to familiarity, and from familiarity into friendship. It was a process, but Brady finally had his first true friend.

When we moved to the specialized school in second grade, Brady and Cody had to part ways. Once again Brady would be alone, and once again, I worried. Neurotypical kids seemed to make friends in an instant. My friend's daughter would meet another child on the playground and within minutes they would be holding hands and asking the moms for a playdate. That was never the case with Brady. He had never initiated or nurtured a new friendship on his own.

But Brady's new school was small, and the teachers were trained to facilitate social interactions between the students in real time. I prayed the personal, focused attention would turn Brady's book smarts about social cues into street smarts.

A few weeks after school started, a new student joined the class. I was pleasantly surprised when Brady told me about the "new kid," even more so that Brady knew his name! It was a promising social step, which became a giant leap when Brady told me he wanted to make friends with him. My heart jumped.

He *wanted* it. That was new, and that was the holy grail of social development. All the interventions and therapies over the years provided Brady with paper knowledge about friendships. They could even help him be more accepted with others, but until he wanted a new friend, he couldn't make one. This was the first time he was introduced to a new child, liked him, and wanted to pursue a relationship. This was big.

Brady was so excited after the first few times they played together he told me he wanted to write a theme song for their friendship. I encouraged him to tone his enthusiasm down just a bit—we didn't want to scare him off! But inside I was writing my own song. I was elated that my son was finally coming out of his cocoon.

Over the next couple of years his desire for friends continued to grow, thanks to the nurturing environment of his specialty schools. He had a small circle of boys he enjoyed, and while he still preferred kids with neurodiversity, he was learning valuable lessons in safe environments about building and maintaining relationships.

In fifth grade, we moved Brady back to a private Christian school. It was a big risk, both socially and academically, and I won't lie, the first couple weeks were tough. Brady loved his teacher and the school itself, but he was having a hard time finding kids to play with at recess.

One morning the parents were invited to a flag raising ceremony on the playground before school. I was standing with Brady when I saw another boy pulling his mom by the arm, marching toward Brady and me like he was on a mission. The boy swung the woman around to face me and said, "Mom, this is Brady's Mom. Get her number. We're having a playdate." I looked over at Brady and his face lit up like a Christmas tree. His shoulders went up an inch and I could see him trying unsuccessfully to suppress a smile that seemed to want to burst from his cheeks. I felt the same way. Owen became Brady's best friend, and they are two peas in a pod to this day. To loosely quote *Casablanca,* it was the beginning of a beautiful friendship.

Brady still struggles in social situations, and probably always will. Since he started middle school the complexity factor jumped to an eleven out of ten. It's a progressive learning curve that seems to steepen exponentially. It currently resembles the warp wall in *American Ninja Warrior.*

My biggest concern about Brady's future isn't related to academics or accomplishment, but the protection of his heart. The boy who didn't recognize the social cues from Justin in the pool is gone. Brady is fully aware of his uniqueness, and has suffered bullying, loneliness, and insecurity at the hands of other kids who are cruel and uncompassionate. This is why it is so important for me to ensure Brady knows his identity in Christ. He is fearfully and wonderfully made. He was made on purpose for a purpose, and God doesn't make mistakes.

Brady's default response to social difficulties is to isolate, just like I did at the beginning of our KIND journey. But God's solution is community. And the friends He carefully and intentionally places in our lives are the sweetest, KIND-est reminder I know of how completely God loves us.

PART 3:

ACCEPTiNG

"You can't go back and change the beginning, but you can start where you are and change the ending."
—C.S. Lewis

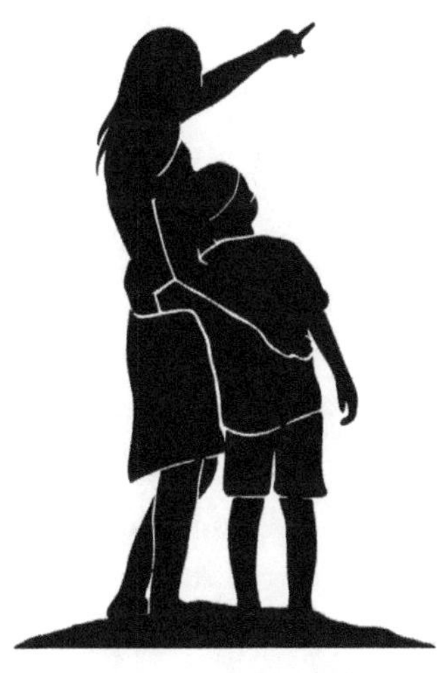

CHAPTER 15
i HAVE FiRE

As I mentioned before, John and I were not church members when Brady was born, so we did not get him baptized right away. However, soon after Brady's autism diagnosis I started having major anxiety about his future. Not just his earthly future; whether he could be independent, hold a job, or get married, although those concerns kept me up at night as well. No, these fears were fueled by the fire of world events that had a whiff of the apocalypse, and I felt a visceral, unexplainable urgency to get him baptized. If the end of the world was really coming, I wanted his soul to be saved, even though I didn't really know what that meant. In my mind it was better to be safe than sorry.

Brady was attending a Lutheran preschool, so we knew he was getting a daily dose of Jesus and the Bible. But I wasn't sure if his special brain could accept something like faith. He had a very literal, black-and-white view of the world, and if something wasn't tangible, visible, and easily understandable, it wasn't real. But I was determined to get Brady baptized anyway.

I found out many churches wouldn't perform baptisms on kids Brady's age. It was either a baby sprinkle or an adult dunk—nothing in between. Fortunately, the pastor at his preschool agreed Brady could be baptized during one of the contemporary Megalife services. Since I didn't really understand baptism, it didn't matter to me where we took Brady for the ritual. If there had been a drive-through option, I would have been fine with it.

Once we had the date scheduled, we invited friends and family to the service and planned a celebration lunch afterward. The morning of the service, John, Brady and I all joined the pastor on the steps of the stage, facing a large congregation. We hadn't rehearsed the sequence of events, so I was surprised when Pastor Jeremy handed our severely uncoordinated four-year-old son a lit candle to hold during his remarks. I quickly pivoted so I could stand behind Brady and put my hands on either side of his, praying we wouldn't burn down the sanctuary. Brady didn't hear a word the pastor said about the sacrament of baptism, and frankly neither did I. I kept my focus on the candle, trying to prevent a four-alarm fire. Brady just stared into the flame with wide eyes and a huge grin. Finally, he couldn't contain his joy any longer. He lifted his gaze into the crowd, found my sister in the audience and yelled, "Auntie Kimberly, I have FIRE!!"

Thankfully the ceremony concluded, and we didn't burn down the church. In my mind Brady's eternity was finally secure. I had checked the box and could relax. My flawed perception of baptism gave me the false confidence that when John, Brady and I met St. Peter at the Pearly Gates he would glance at his clipboard, see we had completed the prerequisites and open the doors.

Obviously I was lacking a true sense of what it means to be a Christ follower. In hindsight it's almost comical that I thought a little water on Brady's head would make the difference between spending eternity in heaven or hell. As if he was suddenly bulletproof. I didn't realize baptism was just a symbolic, outward act, but the real change had to be internal and complete. My heart needed a makeover, but I certainly never considered a do-over to my own "check the box" baptism in high school thirty years earlier.

Over the next couple of years, as my faith grew, Brady was also showing signs of a belief in God that was mature beyond his age. He loved his Bible lessons at school, and was asking me questions that were deep and thoughtful, many beyond my ability to answer. I was hopeful he would find a way to convince his very black-and-white brain that he could have faith in something he could not see and could never fully understand.

One night in first grade Brady walked into the family room with his children's Bible. He opened it to the illustration of Jesus on the cross, set it down, and said forcefully, "I don't believe this." My heart sank, and I feared this was the moment he would reject Jesus outright. I put my poker face on and asked him which part he didn't believe. Brady replied, "That he came back from the dead." Well, shoot. The resurrection is pretty much in the top three of the concepts you need to believe to be a Christian.

I took a deep breath and told Brady that Jesus was a real person, and there is historical evidence of his life and crucifixion. But, it was up to him to decide if he believes Jesus is the son of God, and that he rose from the dead to save us. He looked at me for a few moments, then turned around and walked toward the sliding door. It was dark outside so I asked what he was doing, and he said, "I'm going to pray." Keep in mind, he was six. How does a child that young have the spiritual foundation to take his questions directly to God? I was floored.

He walked into the backyard, turned around, closed the door (a shocker in itself), walked to our firepit and sat down with his back to me. I flipped around and hit my knees so fast I almost crushed our dog sleeping beneath me. I prayed out loud for Brady to hear God at that moment. For God to help him believe.

Brady finally came inside after about ten minutes and nonchalantly said, "It's okay, Mommy. I believe now." When he started to walk back to his room, I breathed a heavy sigh and fought back tears as I asked him what changed his mind. He said, "God told me it was true."

Talk about an answered prayer. God had that one on express delivery. Amazon Prime would be envious of his turnaround time. But hang on, it gets better. Once Brady closed his door and I knew he was out of earshot I cried and thanked God out loud for His Voice and His Presence.

A few minutes later, still in wonder but not knowing what to do with myself in the silence, I picked up my phone. When I opened Facebook the very first post was a Bible verse on a plain turquoise background. It was Psalm 66:19 (HCSB), "However,

God has listened; He has paid attention to the sound of my prayer." My knees just about gave out and I had to lean my elbows on the counter, resting my head in my hands. I knew God could use anything for good, but Facebook? It was like God wanted to assure me that He'd closed the deal. Brady's brain isn't supposed to be wired for faith, but God got him there. It makes sense, since God made his brain, He would know how to reach Brady, and when.

If you aren't sure if faith is possible for yourself or a loved one, just know that God has an infinite toolbox of strategies to get you there. Brady needed to hear God's voice, so he spoke. But sometimes it's more subtle. Sometimes it's an unexplainable peace that comes over you in the middle of a storm. Sometimes it's a compilation of scenarios that could have only come together with Divine intervention. Or sometimes, like in my case, He meets you in the darkness of your circumstances with His Word. Wherever you are, He'll meet you there too.

A couple of years later, our church started advertising upcoming baptism services. By this time Brady was nine, and they opened it up to kids in his grade. I was more than a little surprised when he said he wanted to be baptized again.

At our church, baptisms were a long way from the "sprinkle" service for babies I was used to as a former Presbyterian. Believers profess their belief in Christ and their desire to follow Him through full immersion into a lukewarm tub on stage in front of the whole congregation, while a worship band plays in the background. To be honest, public baptisms initially made me uncomfortable, like worshipers with hands in the air. But I always found it to be a powerful display of faith, and I was usually in tears as I watched people spring out of the water with the energy of new life.

I played the mom card with Brady and said "We'll see," which every kid recognizes as a euphemism for "No." I knew he loved the Lord and learning about the Bible, but he seemed young to take that kind of step. Plus, the kid was a magnet to a microphone or a stage (like his mama), so I was afraid he wanted to do it for attention, not as a statement of faith. I had a business trip scheduled for the weekend the baptisms were to take place, so it bought me some time. I told Brady we could talk about it next time around and figured he would forget all about it.

As it turns out, everyone who wanted to be baptized that April had to forget about it thanks to the Covid shutdown, but later that year as the world started to reopen, the church announced baptisms would happen again in late November. Brady had not forgotten, and asked again if he could be baptized.

This time I called the youth pastor, Lori, and she offered to get on a Zoom call with both of us to discuss it. I sat next to Brady during the call and was amazed at the maturity and awareness of the answers he gave her about his faith. He talked about what it means to be baptized, why he wanted to get baptized, and why he thought it would change his life forever. At nine, he was further in his understanding of baptism than I had been just a few years earlier. I thought back to that moment when God spoke to him. I had no choice but to support him after that conversation.

Just as we were about to hang up, Brady said, "Mom, why don't you get baptized with me?" I blurted out an awkward laugh, waiting for Lori to laugh too. But she didn't. She just smiled and raised her eyebrow. I entertained the idea for a split second but then quickly shut it down. This was about Brady, not me. Plus, I figured he would not want to share the stage with his mom. But when I looked into his eyes again, he was beaming even brighter, "Would you, Mom?" I paused as my heart flipped, but I still resisted.

"Honey, I've already been baptized." The pastor chimed in with a twinkle in her eye, "So has Brady. There's no rule that says you can't do it again." My mind raced a few more seconds before I looked at Brady and asked, "Would you really want me to?" He answered "Oh, yes, PLEASE do it with me Mom! Please! This could be your do-over since your first baptism wasn't special!" I wanted to give them both another excuse, but this time the Holy Spirit wouldn't let me put it off. I suddenly knew there was no other way to respond but "Yes."

***

I realize many of you reading this may not have faith, and a baptism story may not resonate with you. But this isn't just about baptism. It's about never underestimating what God can do with your life, even if your original plan is torn to shreds. Unfortunately, when we are faced with a reality that doesn't follow our desired script, many of us abandon constructive activities and just keep planning: planning for pain, planning for struggle, and planning for disappointment.

But your story is still in progress, and if you let God be the Author, anything is possible. Remember, He is the Creator of creativity, and He is full of surprises. I can attest to that.

On paper, Brady shouldn't believe in God. On paper, Brady shouldn't have friends. On paper, Brady shouldn't be excelling in school. But what is on paper is not the final word for God. He can work in us and through us to produce results you could never predict, using methods you would never expect, and in places you would never imagine. Even Facebook.

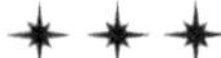

A few weeks later Brady and I were dressed in our matching blue T-shirts and swim bottoms. The room went dark as the video of our pre-baptism interviews filled the large screen over the stage.

Brady and I had been filmed the week before, answering questions about why we wanted to get baptized. Brady brought the house down when he answered, "Well, I have been baptized before, but only because my mom forced me to . . ." The crowd laughed heartily but got quiet as he talked about how he used to be afraid at night, but when he started praying to God the fear went away.

My response was short and sweet. God had revealed himself to me in so many ways by making me Brady's mom. I wanted to be baptized because Brady made me understand baptism wasn't about checking a box, it was about wanting the world to know that my heart had been changed, and I had given it to Jesus.

When the video ended, Brady and I were standing waist deep in the dark tub of lukewarm water with Pastor Lori. The band started to play, and I went first. Lori put her arm around me and asked me if I accepted Jesus as my Lord and Savior. I sputtered out a yes that sounded more like a half cry, she placed her hand behind my back and lowered me gently into the water.

I know I was only under the surface for a moment, but it felt longer. When the water enveloped me, it was as if my past was released into the darkness, disappearing, evaporating in its warmth. I rose up out of the quiet tub into the roaring cheers and strains of pounding worship music, and I was new. I was filled. I was whole.

Then it was Brady's turn. Lori whispered in his ear for a few moments and with him cradled in her arms she leaned him backwards into the water. I will never forget his face when he emerged—it was pure joy. We squeezed each other tightly like we were the only ones in the room.

Finally, I understood baptism. It's the sweetest surrender to a new life, not a box to be checked. When I forced Brady to get baptized the first time, I was trying to force a false salvation on my son because I didn't believe that he could have it for himself. I put God in a box, a box that I tried to "check" myself, assuming He couldn't break through and reach Brady. Boy, was I wrong.

This time we both had fire. The Holy Spirit kind.

CHAPTER 16
CAVERS AND MULES

I have been blessed with a flexible work schedule since I became a mom. I owned my consulting practice so I could block out periods of time during the day for shuttling Brady around town, or if there were special events I wanted to attend. This allowed me to volunteer as a chaperone for almost every one of Brady's field trips with school.

In all honesty, my motivation to accompany Brady and his classmates off campus was not a pure heart for service. Field trips were wild cards for Brady. He always attended small schools, so they didn't have buses, and anything off campus usually required parent drivers. He was not a fan of driving in general, and I imagined long stretches in a stranger's car might result in a tough journey for the chauffeur.

If he made it to the destination unscathed, I was concerned about him running away. Escaping is common for someone with autism, and when Brady was faced with a fight or flight response, he would flee. It was also important for me to see him interact socially with his peers, and if possible, to intervene in the moment to help him better relate to his classmates.

But as Brady got older these special outings became easier. He looked forward to escaping the classroom, and his tendency to run away waned. He also started to make some friends and develop some independence. I started to wonder how much longer he was going to want his mom tagging along.

In the spring of sixth grade, Brady's science teacher announced a day-long trip to Kartchner Caverns and Bisbee Mines in Southeastern Arizona. This was a time commitment far beyond the regular school day, and I silently prayed this would be the trip for him to spread his wings and go without me. Alas, the school needed extra drivers, and I was on the list.

Door to door it was about 450 miles of driving in a single day. We had to meet at his school at 6:00 a.m., and we live 30 minutes away, so it was still dark when we left the house. I brought a giant mug full of double-strength coffee to urge my sleepy eyes to stay awake. Brady didn't need a caffeine jolt—he was excited for the adventure, especially since his best friend, Owen, was assigned to our car.

Our house is a straight shot on the same road from our neighborhood exit to the school parking lot. That morning the full moon was setting directly in front of us against a dark periwinkle sky. The farther we drove the larger it appeared as it fell from its perch, until it looked like we would be swallowed up by the yellow glow at the end of the horizon. I'm not superstitious, but it wasn't lost on me that chaperoning a bunch of sixth graders across the state during a full moon might present some challenges.

We arrived at school and joined the other families to await instructions from the teacher. She handed the drivers manila folders, like she was the handler giving us a top-secret mission. Inside the folder were directions, addresses, rules of the road, and copies of the permission slips for my passengers.

After a quick group prayer we loaded into our cars. The first leg was about three hours, and I was able to use the time to catch up on podcasts and audiobooks, while my son and his friend watched movies on the iPad.

Oh, how much easier life would have been with the iPad in the car when Brady was younger! All we had was a portable DVD player, and it presented almost as many problems as solutions. We traveled with a black zip up case with about 30 disk sleeves inside. Brady would select the show he wanted to watch before we left the house, but it would inevitably skip, or he would get tired of one DVD and demand another. I would wind up doing Cirque du Soleil acrobatics to keep one foot on the gas and one hand on the steering wheel while I reached with the other arm behind my headrest to remove the player from the straps so I could change the movie. I admit, those were not some of my shining moments as a responsible driver.

We arrived at Kartchner Caverns around 9:30 a.m. Brady and his friend jumped out of the car and sprinted straight for the visitor's center gift shop. Brady has always had an insatiable need to purchase large quantities of worthless, overpriced junk whenever possible, so we spent the next 10 minutes negotiating which treasures he could afford and could not live without.

We explored the museum as we waited for our guided tour to start. One display explained how the caverns were discovered. About fifty years ago, a cave enthusiast named Randy Tufts, who also happened to be a PhD, geologist, and planetary scientist, was on a lunch date and came across a small crack at the bottom of a sinkhole in the earth. Randy spent his youth exploring caves ravaged by vandalism, and his lifelong dream was to find an undiscovered cave and preserve it for visitors for years to come.

Randy returned to the sinkhole with his friend and fellow caver Gary Tenen, they geared up and squeezed themselves into the opening. They shimmied on their bellies in the narrow hole for the length of a football field! When they reached the end of the tunnel, they found a small bat hole and smelled bat guano. Instead of turning back, they started chipping away at the hole with their tools. What lay before them was a gigantic cave filled with stalactites and stalagmites that looked like something out of a science fiction movie.

Our tour guides pointed out the sinkhole as we rode in the electric trams up a windy cement road to the entrance to the cave. After disembarking we gathered around for quick instructions before we entered. The guides told us that if any part of our clothing, shoes, or skin touched the walls of the cave, we needed to let them know so they could tag the location for sanitation later. I figured that might be an issue for Brady and told him he needed to be extra careful, and he replied with a middle-school-sized eye roll.

The guides opened the door, which looked like it belonged to a blast-proof bank vault, and we entered the dimly lit hallway. Ahead of us was a narrow cement path, and the air was damp and cool. We passed under the spray of a mister which was intended to reduce the amount of lint we carried in on our clothes. It also served to frizz my hair.

Wide smiles covered the boys' faces as they skipped down the walkway with their heads pivoting left and right. After a few minutes walking down a mild grade we turned a corner, and we could see our first glimpse of the rough, icicle-like structures hanging from the ceiling and the finger-like growths coming out of the ground.

The guides kept us moving while they shared informative facts mixed with a family friendly comedy routine. They let us stop occasionally as they explained the geological origins of the stalactites, stalagmites, and my personal favorite—"bacon"—formations throughout the caves. Brady stopped frequently to raise his hand and confess that a foot or hand had accidentally touched the surface. A mama knows. The kind guides took it in stride, marked the spots with a red ribbon and moved on. Brady listened intently and stayed with the class.

We ended the tour in the "Throne Room." There were three rows of stone, amphitheater-style benches, positioned toward the expansive cave. We all took a seat, and Brady slid up close to my side, so I put my arms around him, hoping the move wouldn't embarrass him in front of his classmates. It didn't. Soft violin music began to fill the room, and in a choreographed flow, light started to illuminate the magical formations one by one. As we watched and listened, I thought about the day so far and marveled not just at the geological wonder in front of me, but at the young man next to me and how far he had come since those early field trips. I had time to consider the majesty of the moment, and the parallels of my story to Randy's and Gary's started to crystallize. Maybe you can relate.

Anytime you deal with a life challenge, whether a diagnosis for yourself or your child, or any other setback, it can feel like you are threading yourself through a small opening, with no wiggle room or fresh air to breathe. The walls seem like they are pressing in on you, and you wonder if you will ever find the wide-open space you once enjoyed before entering the hole. But eventually, if you keep crawling through, even at a snail's pace, there is a light at the end of the tunnel. It might even seem like a dead end, and it may smell like bat guano, but you hold your breath and keep punching through. Your reward may be even more than the space you crave, it could be a wonderful discovery of God's glory that was just temporarily hidden from view.

We only had a few minutes to sit and contemplate our surroundings and their metaphorical application to our lives before they herded us back outside to the tram. By the time we left the visitor's center it was almost lunchtime, and we had to hustle back in the car to travel another hour to Bisbee for our next stop.

Bisbee is a famous old mining town not far from the real O.K. Corral. We arrived to find a town built on a hillside to our left, and the rickety mine shaft to our right. We entered the visitor's center and hit the gift shop once again, but this time Brady resisted the urge to add to his collection.

When they called our group for the tour, we were all given construction vests, hard hats, and a heavy lamp with a battery that we wore around our necks. I grimaced at the thought of wearing the same helmet on my head as hundreds of other visitors, but Brady and his friend embraced the costume and twirled the lamps around like a lasso.

According to our guide, the mine was opened in the late 1800s and the shaft we entered through started production in 1915. The train we boarded to enter the cool, dark narrow cave looked like it went into service on day one. It was a simple design with five or six segments. Each "car" had a long plank of wood for the seat with parallel foot guards on either side below. The visitors straddled the board, all sitting facing the same direction with their knees bent so that we looked like a set of nesting dolls. My nose was inches from the sweaty shirt of the chaperone in front of me, and my son wrapped his arms around my waist like we were heading out on the open road on a Harley. Instead, we were rolling 1,500 feet into the side of the mountain.

Deep inside the old mine shaft we exited the train and started walking through the dark and dusty cave. Our guide, who looked like a genuine prospector himself, explained how they blasted with dynamite drilled deep into holes in the rock. The heavy ore was sent down chutes from higher levels of the mine into huge metal tubs sitting on the tracks. He told us that for the first couple of decades of the mine's operation, men had to push the cars full of tons of rock back out of the shaft to be processed. Brady and I exchanged glances in silent agreement—that would not have been a fun job!

Finally, the tour guide explained, someone had the idea that they could use mules to pull the carts, which would save time and some of the physical toll the hard labor was causing their workers. The mine operators brought the mules into the mines where they stayed in service underground for four to five years, never leaving the dark confines of their worksite. They had their own stables, good food and water, and on-site veterinarian care. The mules adapted well to their new environment, and their contribution improved the efficiency and safety of the mine tremendously. It was the next part of the story that intrigued me the most.

When the mules' tour of duty in the mine came to an end, the veterinarians knew that if they were exposed to direct sunlight after years of living in darkness, it could blind them permanently. So, they led the pack out of the caves at night and brought them into a barn nearby that had been completely sealed from any natural light. Every door and window were covered so it was completely dark except for a dim lantern that mimicked the environment from which they had come.

Then, each day, someone would adjust the barn window ever so slightly. Each day, they continued to widen the opening in the window just a smidgen more until finally the warmth and glow of the midday sun could fill the barn. When their eyes were fully adjusted, they were finally released to breathe the clean, crisp air of the outdoors.

Here I was again, with a vivid picture in my head, and this time, I was the mule. You see, I was in the figurative dark for years after we realized Brady had autism. My grief over the loss of what I perceived to be a typical parenting experience combined with Brady's uncertain future applied a layer of heaviness that kept me from the joy that was available to me. I'm sure you have been through a season like that in your life—one that temporarily overpowered the light in your life. If you are in that place now, you may have even forgotten what it was like before the light was taken away.

As I started leaning into faith a few years after Brady's diagnosis, I could look back and see God at work everywhere. He let a little bit of light in each day, so this stubborn mule gradually started to understand how to live out of the darkness. I found Jesus in the light, and once I could see the light, I could be the light for others.

On the long car ride back home, I considered the day and thanked God again for His provision (and for the iPad to entertain the boys). Brady rocked the field trip. We had come so far since those early days when I would have been running after him or nervously monitoring his interactions all day. More than any other excursion, I was able to enjoy the sites and my son at the same time.

As the sun set in the distance, it streaked the sky with blazing red and orange grandeur, and even as darkness fell, I could still see the light.

CHAPTER 17
THE POWER OF A T-SHiRT

Sports and fitness have always been an important part of my life. I snow skied from an early age, and I even won a first-place trophy for a ski race when I was about seven years old. Admittedly, my speed was due to my desperate need for a potty break. I tucked into a ball as I barreled down the hill to the bathrooms. The strategy apparently helped me outpace the more upright, bladder-controlled competitors.

I played golf and softball through junior high, and some tennis and volleyball in high school. If you will allow me a brief Al Bundy "glory days" moment, even though I'm only 5'3" on a good hair day, I made the All-City volleyball team as a setter my senior year.

I had a short-lived love affair with running in my twenties, mostly because it helped me metabolize the happy hour buffets I was frequenting, but after a knee injury I resorted to other low-impact ways to stay in shape.

Somehow the sports gene fell off the strand of DNA on its way to Brady. One of the side effects of Brady's autism is low muscle tone, balance issues, and a lack of coordination that comes from not knowing where his body is in space. That makes most sports difficult for him, especially those involving balls. I remember during one physical therapy evaluation, the provider threw a soft squishy ball at Brady's face, and he didn't even flinch as it hit him square in the nose.

That is not to say we didn't try. We had a t-ball set in the backyard, but Brady would only hit a few Wiffle balls before he was done. John told him to keep his eye on the ball, and Brady dutifully walked over and placed his actual eye on the actual ball.

John tried to play "catch" with him, and it was more like "throw and pick up." We tried playing soccer with him and even signed him up for a basketball team, but Brady quickly caught on that both sports were really running in disguise. Brady hated running. At one summer sports camp the counselors made the kids run around the gym if they weren't listening. Brady deemed that "torture" and was mad about it for days.

Brady was a self-described "indoor kid." His favorite hobbies were reading, watching the iPad, and playing video games, none of which provided the physical activity he needed as a growing boy. I worried about his health, and longed for him to know what it feels like to be in good physical shape and to be part of a team.

The only outdoor activity he ever enjoyed was swimming. He loved being submerged in the pool. As a sensory seeker the pressure of the water touching every part of his body was calming to him. But if a pool was not nearby, the only way to get him to exercise was to withhold screentime until he performed some minimal activity like jumping jacks or pushups.

I knew only an act of God could reverse his aversion to exercise. Or a T-shirt. That kid would do anything for a T-shirt. But I prayed earnestly for a fitness awakening.

About a month into fifth grade, Brady switched schools. He moved to a small school with a focus on participation, not performance, so he could be part of a sports team without fear of getting cut. Because we missed the first part of the school year, the swim team had already been practicing for several weeks, and it was too late to join. When Brady noticed that the kids on the swim team got to wear jeans and swim team T-shirts instead of the formal school uniform on meet days, he vowed to join the team the following year. That is, of course, if we promised to buy him one of the shirts.

At the beginning of sixth grade, Brady stayed true to his word and said he wanted to join the swim team. Practices were three days a week and didn't start until 5:00 p.m., which meant Brady and I would have to kill a couple hours after school, then get home late and deal with homework. I was nervous about how Brady would handle the taxing schedule, and how I would handle the probable fallout. Ultimately, John and I decided the exercise alone was worth it. Brady would also learn valuable lessons about time management, organization, and pushing himself to function when he was tired. The positives outweighed the negatives, and we registered Brady for his inaugural school sport.

However, the first practice was almost his last. Since Brady was new to competitive swimming, the coach placed in a swim lane with the fifth graders, not the other sixth grade boys in his class. She moved him down so he could get more basic instruction on the strokes, but Brady was devastated, and from my seat at the edge of the pool I could see a storm brewing behind his eyes.

Within seconds Brady's emotions bubbled into a full fight or flight response. He pulled himself out of the pool and bolted to the parking lot in bare feet, soaking wet and shirtless. I ran after him, grateful for the cement wall that blocked us from the team's view. I tried to calmly explain the reason for the coach's actions and begged him to get back in the pool. Brady refused and continued to inch toward the car. This was a sad moment in full swing.

After several minutes of pleading unsuccessfully with Brady to finish practice, I finally relented and said we could go. But on the way to the car, I told Brady how proud I was that he'd been brave enough to join the team in the first place. Suddenly Brady flinched. "You were proud of me?" he asked. I nodded, "Very."

I could see Brady's face start to soften, and his resolve start to waver, so I asked him one more time to return to practice. I threw in a promise of a spaghetti dinner for good measure, and this time he agreed.

I may not have tried so hard to convince Brady to stay on the swim team had I ever attended a swim meet before. Swim meets in Arizona are painfully long and occur during the hottest part of the year. John and I would set up camp with the other parents, chasing whatever shade we could find in the triple-digit temps. We would pack coolers with frozen water bottles, cold towels, and plenty of Gatorade and sunscreen.

Remember those soccer moms, whose weekend sports schedules prompted me to pray for a kid who loved to read? This was my payback. At least those moms got to watch their kid perform for more than two minutes.

Throughout the season, Brady continued to improve. His goal at each meet was to get a PR (personal record) and he almost always did. The rush of shaving seconds off his time and the support of his teammates gave him confidence and pride, in a way he'd never experienced before. Brady found his sport. He was a swimmer.

That year, the State Swim Meet was open to almost everyone, and Brady got to compete in his favorite event, the 50-yard freestyle. The energy at the evening championship was electric. Brady felt the excitement of the competition, and he stayed engaged and playful with his teammates while he waited for his event. When it was go-time, John and I hugged him tightly and told him to do his best, but emphasized we were proud of him no matter what. We knew he wanted to finish the season with a PR, and felt he had a good chance to succeed.

The gun went off, Brady dove into the water, and when his head came up, his goggles came down off his eyes. I felt a stabbing pain in my heart. He would be disqualified if he touched them, but even if he didn't, the possibility of a PR was slim.

But Brady didn't stop. He pulled hard with his arms and kicked violently with his feet, disregarding the goggles which settled just above his upper lip. When he made the turn, he got a great push off the wall and kept going. We cheered wildly even though we knew he couldn't hear us. And when he touched the other edge of the pool I looked up at the scoreboard. He had taken almost five seconds off his best time ever! He may as well have won the state championship in his mind—and in ours.

Brady taught me lots of lessons during his first swim season. First, sometimes we need to take a step back and humble ourselves in order to move forward. Pride could have kept Brady from getting back in the pool before he even had his first meet, but swimming was something he loved, and he suppressed the need to quit. Secondly, Brady learned he could do hard things. Now the next time he is presented with a challenge, he will remember that he overcame obstacles both physically and mentally in other areas of his life. Plus, swimming planted the seed in Brady's mind that a healthy body is a helpful body. We hoped that seed would grow.

When the swim season was over Brady told me he wanted to join cross-country. I could not have been more stunned. I had to ask him, "Do you know what cross-country is?" I was afraid he thought it was a travel club. He assured me he knew the sport involved running, but based on his vocal hatred of anything that required running in the past, I was skeptical. He told me he really liked the teacher who would be coaching, and of course, there would be another T-shirt. So, we agreed to let him give it a try, after I confirmed with the school that if he quit in the first two weeks we could get our $200 registration fee back.

Practices were right after school and on campus, so from a parenting perspective I knew this would be my favorite sport. I had an extra hour before I had to pick him up at school, and we would get home in time to do homework before Brady's brain transformed into mush. Still, I wondered if he would change his mind about cross-country after a couple of practices during which he would have to actually, you know, run.

He didn't. The coach brilliantly structured the practices to include some form work, some games, and some running, usually to a park or a trailhead nearby. Brady loved going off campus, and never once complained about the practices. He thought they were fun. He even liked the days they had to run up "Heartbreak Hill," the steep desert trail that had a storied history of kids collapsing in tears before reaching the summit.

The team only had a handful of practices before the first meet. A middle-school, cross-country competition is a two-mile course, and on the way to the field Brady revealed he had never run that far. Not in practice, not ever. I prepared myself for the worst, but

I reassured him along with his coaches that it was okay to walk if he got tired. The only goal was to complete the race. I even offered a McDonald's dinner if he made it through the finish line. But honestly, I gave it about a 50/50 chance that he would quit, or that at the end of the race he would tell us he was done with cross-country.

When it came time for the boys to line up, it finally dawned on me that he would disappear around a corner in about 50 yards and I wouldn't be able to see him. The assistant coach had been to the location before and pointed out the best spot for John and me to stand to see him at certain points of the race. I did the only thing I knew—I prayed that God would be with him. I prayed for safety, stamina, and encouragement.

The boys gathered inside a narrow part of the field that had been marked with cones. They were all crammed in together, like sardines in a can. I couldn't see Brady in the middle of all the taller, older boys. After a quick "On your mark," through a megaphone, the gun went off. Instantly the crowd started moving like an amoeba at first, then slowly individual runners started to separate from the pack. I finally caught a glimpse of Brady as most of the kids ran ahead of him. The first thing I noticed was that his shoelace was untied. He had only been running for about 30 seconds, and he already had a challenge to overcome.

A few moments later he disappeared around the corner, and John and I weren't sure what to do. We moved with the other parents to the spot that would offer us the next glimpse of the boys and waited. And waited. It was excruciating, especially as other kids came into view, but Brady did not. Just when I was about to start running in the opposite direction to find him, I could see Brady on the path. He was walking and looked spent, but when he saw John and me and heard us screaming his name, he started running again. The course was a loop, so we had to go through that cycle a few more times. Then, in the final leg of the race, he gave it everything he had and ran full speed through the finish line. He did it! I hugged him so tightly my shirt absorbed his sweat marks. Once again, I underestimated his tenacity.

Later, when we were in the car with a McDonald's shake in hand, I asked him if he really liked running. He replied, "I love it, but not until twenty minutes after I'm done."

Not only did Brady keep running cross-country, but he continued to get personal records in each meet, and within a couple of races, he stopped walking at all. He even started running 5ks, and not just to add to his growing T-shirt collection. Brady proved with each accomplishment he wasn't a quitter; he was an overcomer. He reinvented himself, destroying many of the perceived limitations that had deceived us when he was diagnosed. He discovered a part of his identity that had been there all along. The one with strength and perseverance and courage. The one God gave him.

We are all a work in progress as we try to become firmly rooted in our identity as a child of God. In his second letter to Timothy, Paul tells us that God has not given us a spirit of fear, but one of power, love, and sound judgment. Sometimes a diagnosis or other setback can trick us into placing a false boundary around our expectations. But God doesn't have boundaries. He knows your potential, and if He made you for a purpose beyond that boundary, He will help you jump the fence.

Brady's transformation from couch potato to athlete is a testament to the power of prayer and the power of identity, in Christ. And yes, to the power of a T-shirt.

CHAPTER 18
"DANCiNG QUEEN" & THE LiP-SYNC MACHiNE

I started playing the piano when I was so little I still had to put a phone book on the bench to reach the keys. For those of you a bit younger, a phone book was a large, heavy paperback about four inches tall in which everyone's home phone numbers were listed in alphabetical order. If you don't know what a home phone is, ask your mom.

Everyone knew me as the girl who could play piano, so for choir and church events I usually wound up as the accompanist. But what no one knew was that I really wanted to sing. I spent countless hours in my room with my door closed, wielding a brush like a microphone and entertaining the throngs of fans I imagined were cheering for me inside my mirror. It was usually "Dancing Queen" or some other ABBA album that would bring the house down.

When it came time to choose a major in college, I didn't even consider something like music or the arts. According to my parents, the most logical and responsible major was business, and I agreed. I wanted to make money, and I wanted to be perceived as successful. Starving artist was not the job description that fit into my life plan.

However, when karaoke became popular in my twenties, I got the bug to sing again. My friends and I frequented some bars with karaoke and loved cheering and jeering the brave souls who bared their hearts and voices for a roomful of half-sauced strangers. But

I rarely took the stage unless it was a group effort, and it usually required a few adult beverages to grease the skids.

One weekend I was invited to go on my friend's boat to Catalina Island. We had dinner in a famous restaurant/bar called El Galleon that was known for its karaoke, and my friends started pushing me to sign up. I had been listening to the quality performances and realized the place was out of my league, so I politely declined. I was more comfortable singing as part of an ensemble in the corner of a dive bar where it was dark and late and expectations were low. But this place was packed, with a raised stage, bright lights, and professional acoustics.

Unbeknownst to me, my friends decided to take matters into their own hands. I had just finished my entrée when I heard the DJ exclaim, "Next up we have Kari! Kari, please make your way to the stage!" I glared menacingly at my soon-to-be-former friends as they laughed mischievously and pushed me out of my chair, shoving me toward the stage. I started my slow walk to the front as the audience clapped politely. Then the announcer revealed my song— "Dancing Queen". I panicked. While that song was my all-time favorite and was known as my signature song among close friends, it had some high notes that I conveniently avoided when I sang in my car.

I took the microphone and silently vowed to never speak to my friends again as the music started. Then something magical happened. I started singing, and when I heard my voice over the sound system, it sounded pretty good. By the time I was through the first verse, people started to pay attention, and a few got up from their table and started dancing in front of me. When I hit the refrain "You can dance, you can jive, having the time of your life," it seemed the whole place was filled with smiling faces bouncing, swaying, and singing along. I realized I really was having the time of my life. I was that little girl again, but this time I wasn't imagining the audience—they were real!

I felt a rush like never before, and for the first time questioned my life choices as a finance major. Could I have made it as a singer instead of being a stockbroker? Now, mind you, the cheers of the audience were likely just as much a result of stiff drinks and a great song as my vocal talents, but the damage was done. I would never forget that feeling.

Back at my table, I quickly came back down to earth and abandoned the idea of quitting my job to become a bar singer. I filed the feeling away under the "shoulda coulda" heading and made peace with my life choices. I proudly wore the nickname "Karaoke Kari," however, and even sang "Dancing Queen" at my own wedding. I never forgot what it felt like, but I had no idea how I could make singing a part of my very logical, rational life. It just wasn't part of the plan.

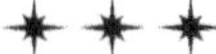

Brady wound up with lots of good qualities from John's side of the family, but there is one deeply ingrained part of Brady's personality that is most definitely, 100 percent from me. His love of the stage. John never liked being in the spotlight, but Brady and I have an unexplainable desire to seek it. The kindergarten talent show was just the beginning for him. He performed solos at Christmas shows, monologues in community plays, and speeches at school competitions. He never shows the slightest bit of fear when asked to perform, and his brain is a steel trap when it comes to memorizing lines. On stage he is at home, confident, and natural.

Last winter, Brady attended our church's Winter Camp at Lost Canyon, a Younglife camp in Williams, Arizona. If you are not familiar with Arizona, it may surprise you to know that just a couple hours north of the hot desert of Phoenix there are evergreen trees, mountains, creeks, and lakes. The climate in Williams is more like Colorado than Arizona, and that winter the region had record snow.

I went along as a member of the work crew, a glorified name for kitchen help. Our job was serving campers their meals and snacks, setting up and clearing tables, scraping food, washing dishes, vacuuming the floor, and any other physical labor that was required to keep over 600 people fed for 48 hours.

I'm not sure I have ever been more physically and mentally exhausted in my life. Friday night the kids had a nacho party at

11:00 p.m., and our cleanup duties kept us out until 1:00 a.m. On Saturday, we were up at 6:00 a.m. to set up breakfast. My health tracking app registered 31,000 steps by dinnertime. We only got a couple of short breaks during the day and all I wanted to do that night was faceplant on any flat surface I could find.

I only saw Brady briefly during the day, but he told me he had signed up for the lip-sync contest later that night. I wasn't surprised. Not only was it a chance to perform, but there was a real-life trophy for the winner. The only thing better than a T-shirt to Brady, is a trophy. He didn't even have to tell me which song he would perform. I knew.

Brady is fascinated with the viral social media phenomenon called "Rickrolling." For those of you not familiar with middle school pranks, it involves sending someone a video link that looks like one thing, but when the person clicks play, they are surprised by the cheesy 80s music video for Rick Astley's "Never Gonna Give You Up." Brady was a master Rickroller, and his victims were many. He even Rickrolled his entire school over the loudspeaker while making the announcements one morning. He was a legend.

The contest didn't start until 10:00 p.m. I was so tired I knew even my snoring bunkmates wouldn't keep me up, but something inside me kept pressing me to go. Those Holy Spirit nudges are especially pesky when they interfere with much-needed sleep. A work crew friend who also had a daughter performing a song in the contest convinced me we shouldn't miss the show. I brushed my teeth and put on my pajamas so I could collapse into bed as soon as it was over, and we threw on our coats and boots and trudged through the snow to the meeting hall.

The contest was held in an old theater-style room packed with rowdy teens and tweens. The stage was like the one from T*he Muppet Show*, with long dark red velour curtains draped across the top and hanging down the sides. I could see Brady in the crowd but kept my distance as the show started. Some of the acts seemed professional, with choreography and ventriloquist-level lip-syncing. Brady's was a cheeky farce. Familiar dread started to flow through me. Were these kids going to be supportive or vicious?

Then the emcee called Brady's name, and something utterly shocking happened. The crowd started chanting his name, "Brady! Brady!" A sly smile came across my son's face as he jumped up and started pushing through the bodies to get to the stage. It took him a minute because kids were high-fiving him and patting his back, and the chanting only got louder as he got closer to the stage. I was stunned. Sure, there were quite a few kids from our church who knew Brady. I assumed some of them knew of his autism, so I expected them to be kind. But most of the campers were from other churches and had no idea who he was.

When the musical intro started, something even more magical happened. Everybody in the room jumped to their feet and started singing along. Brady performed his signature moves and mouthed the words "never gonna give you up, never gonna let you down" with emotion and dramatic flair. He rolled his hips. He circled his arms. He dropped to his knees, Elvis-style. He had no fear. He was in his element. He soaked in the accolades and didn't back off until the music finally faded out, and the crowd went wild. I looked around in disbelief. Everyone was in love with my son.

Once he took his bow the chants started again, "Brady! Brady! Brady!" He had to fight to make his way back up to his seat. One of the male counselors came up to me with tears in his eyes. "I think that is the bravest thing I've ever seen someone do," he told me. He was right.

After all the acts were done, the emcee asked the crowd to pick the winner based on applause, and no one else even had a chance. Brady was the winner by a landslide. I will never forget him holding that trophy over his head like he just won a world championship boxing match as the audience lost their minds.

Watching him perform, I could tell he felt that same stirring I had on stage so many years ago in Catalina. When you use a gift God gave you, your soul fills to the top with joy and starts to pour over. I committed at that moment to help Brady find his passion. Help him use his gifts. Help him fulfill his purpose using the unique set of talents and abilities that could only come from God.

There is no better feeling than finding and acting on your purpose. Fortunately I had a second chance to find mine.

One Sunday our church was making a pitch for volunteers, and one of the options in the bulletin was to join the worship team, which is the rock-style band that performs music at services. John leaned over, pointed at it, shrugged his shoulder, and winked at me, insinuating I should try out. He knew I loved to sing, considering my "Dancing Queen" serenade at our wedding. I almost laughed out loud, shook my head, and gave him my best eye roll so he was sure I thought it was a crazy idea. But the seed had been planted, and after staring at an email to our worship pastor for hours, I finally hit "send" and asked about auditioning as a backup vocalist.

A week later I was in the church auditorium with Joe and his guitar. The song I chose was "No Longer Slaves," the same song that brought me to my knees when I finally started giving my heart to the Lord. When I finished, to my surprise, Joe didn't kick me off the stage. We practiced a couple of other songs, and hearing our voices blend together in harmony, praising God, filled me like nothing I'd ever experienced. My "Dancing Queen" high was not even on the same planet. This wasn't about me or my voice, this was about using one of God's gifts for HIS glory. There is no comparison.

Serving as a backup vocalist for the worship team is one of my greatest joys. As I look out into the congregation and encourage them in worship, I feel as if God's presence is flowing through me like a waterfall. This is how God wanted me to use my voice, of that I am certain now. I'll never make a living as a worship leader, but I can't imagine my life without it. I just wish it hadn't taken me most of my life to figure it out.

God made each one of us with different gifts, and He wants us to use them. Those abilities and talents aren't just for our enjoyment; they help us fulfill our purpose. Like mine, your life plan may be perfectly logical, prudent, and financially sound, but if it doesn't allow you to use your gifts, you are missing out on tremendous joy, and possibly tremendous impact.

If you are a KIND parent, it is critical that your child's natural proficiencies and passions are nurtured and reinforced. So many activities are challenging for neurodiverse kids, so emphasizing the skills they enjoy and excel at allows them to shine in a world that often makes them feel deficient. If you haven't noticed an obvious talent yet, keep trying new things! Your child's passion may even lead to a future career.

I realize not all of us can make a living doing what we love, but we might be able to make a *difference* doing what we love. Most gifts don't require a stage and a spotlight. If someone's gifts are more personal and private, that doesn't make them any less important. Your gift could bring people hope, make people laugh, or lead people to Jesus. If you don't discover your gift and how to use it you aren't just shorting yourself, you are shorting the world.

Whatever is inside you was meant to be shared for the good of others, or God wouldn't have put it there. If you haven't found your gifts yet, keep looking. If you are a parent, observe the things that bring your children pure joy and help them develop those skills. Just like Rick Astley, never give up until you find that stirring, then ask God how he wants you to use it. Take it from Karaoke Kari—it's never too late.

CHAPTER 19
WHAT'S iN A NAME?

Titles are important. I remember my first business card that said "Vice President" under my name. It provided professional validation of my achievements, and I couldn't wait to hand it out to whomever would accept it. When I got married, I loved hearing people address me as Mrs. Baker. And when I became a mom, hearing Brady call me Mommy was the best. Until he started saying it incessantly in repetition, but that's another story.

There are lots of instances in the Bible where a character's name changes. It's not just to confuse us, it is a reflection of a transition in identity. Jacob became Israel, Simon Peter became Peter, and most notably, Saul became Paul. Their name changed to reflect their new purpose as followers of God.

I think my mom wanted to have the title "grandmother" about fifteen minutes after I exited the womb. She was born for it. Unable to wait until I was out of high school, she "adopted" the family across the street and became "Grandma Kay" to the baby. I've already told you how she paid for me to join a dating service in my late thirties. She didn't just want me to have a soulmate, she wanted to be a grandmother. She even called our beagle Bailey her "grand dog."

When Mom found out I was pregnant, she was beside herself with joy, and she was certain I was having a girl. She wouldn't even talk about the possibility of a Y chromosome sneaking in. That is, until the ultrasound revealed an extra appendage which confirmed we were indeed having a baby boy. I called her from the doctor's office and said, "It's a boy, Mom!" For a second, I thought I lost the connection because there was no response. Finally, she said, "Well, I'm sure he'll make a great big brother to my granddaughter someday."

The disappointment was momentary, and as my due date approached, she became convinced that a grandson would be much more fun than a granddaughter. She'd already done the "girl" thing with my sister Kimberly and me anyway. This would be a whole new adventure.

My mom has always been cheerful, but when Brady was born she just exuded delight. When I was struggling as a new mom, we called her the baby whisperer. She could lay Brady on her legs and sway gently back and forth and he would instantly go to sleep. She watched him almost every day so I could work and go to meetings. She rocked him, sang to him, and read to him. She started calling him "the best little boy in the whole wide world," and I knew she believed it was true.

My Dad was a little more reserved during my pregnancy. He was excited but worried about me. He told me once that he couldn't let himself relax until he knew I came through the delivery safe and sound. I was his first priority. That is just like my dad. He is the epitome of fierce love—he would do anything for my mom and his girls.

I loved seeing Dad hold Brady as an infant. They would just look at each other intensely, and it was as if they were having a telepathic conversation only the two of them could understand. When Brady began to walk and talk, my dad jumped into his grandpa shoes with both feet. He loved taking Brady on golf cart rides through the neighborhood and reading to him. The only thing we weren't sure about was what to call him. My mom was already Grandma Kay, would he be Grandpa Gary? Grandpa Dorris?

Brady had other ideas for both my parents. When we would visit my parents we would try to get Brady to say Grandma and Grandpa, but gradually we noticed that when he referred to them, it was something different. My mom was "Gra." That made sense, it was a truncated version of grandma, and my mom enjoyed the uniqueness of her new name. But it took us a while to figure out what Brady was calling my Dad. At first, John thought he was saying "Crawdad," but as he was able to articulate it better, we realized it was Dadat. Gra and Dadat stuck, and the new titles came with new personalities, especially for Dad.

My parents were always concerned with health and fitness. So much so, that my sister and I were only allowed one precious box of sugary cereal per year, on our birthdays. I would agonize over the decision—Apple Jacks or Fruit Loops? We had cookies in the house, but they were considered a special treat and we had to get permission before partaking. And once my dad found out how many tablespoons of sugar were in sodas, we were relegated to TaB for a fizzy beverage. I'm sure the chemically treated sweetener was much better for us.

But Gra and Dadat were different from Mom and Dad. Sugar was frequent and abundant. McDonald's was lunch and ice cream was dinner. One time Dad gave Brady a treat when I had specifically asked him not to, and when he apologized he told me sorrowfully, "He asked for it, and I couldn't say no." He couldn't say no? That isn't my dad either. "No" was on regular rotation at our house, especially when I was a teenager.

This Dadat also had a level of patience that miraculously materialized when Brady was born. The same guy who would leave a restaurant if the wait was more than five minutes, could suddenly sit at a computer screen for hours with Brady on his lap, helping him write stories while typing with his two index fingers.

Most importantly, Gra and Dadat were like the KIND SWAT team when Brady was diagnosed. From the moment I took that online test, they supported John and me in every way. They attended parent training sessions to learn how to recognize and respond to Brady's needs. They read our weekly updates and implemented activities based on our developmental focus that week. They babysat Brady to give us much-needed breaks for dinner or even weekends away. They respected the treatment decisions John and I made, and frequently reminded us that we were great parents, even when it felt like the opposite was true. Gra and Dadat made Brady's well-being the center of their lives.

At one point, Dad confessed that he saw a lot of himself in Brady. Right after we told Brady about his diagnosis, he wrote Brady a long letter telling him how he was different as a kid too. He loved to collect and sort hundreds of marbles, he had trouble focusing, he didn't like playing with other kids unless they played something he was interested in. He wrote, " When I was a boy, no one knew about ADHD or autism. People just called us different. I do not know if I have ADHD or if I am autistic. I just know that as a kid I did not think the same way as other kids. And that made me different, but that was OK."

My parents were wonderful human beings before Brady, but as Gra and Dadat, they are superheroes, especially to Brady. Becoming Gra fulfilled my mom's purpose, and becoming Dadat brought new purpose to Dad.

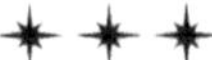

My sister Kimberly is about four years older than me. She received the undivided attention of my parents for her entire young life until I came along, which is documented by multiple volumes of photo albums of her every move. I think she was less than thrilled when I was born and upset her apple cart. I'm sure it was a challenge for my parents as well, as evidenced by the fact that there are only a handful of pictures of me from birth to toddlerhood.

Kimberly is a self-described introvert, and as a kid she was mostly serious, quiet and shy, unless she was around close friends. I was the polar opposite, an extrovert who never missed an opportunity to strike up a conversation with a stranger, or even give an impromptu performance in a crowded restaurant. Throughout our childhood, we struggled to find common ground. Kimberly didn't appreciate my need for attention, and I didn't appreciate her ability to outsmart me. In my defense, mud looks an awful lot like a chocolate shake.

We tried to fight, which probably would have been healthy, but our parents usually nipped it in the bud to try to maintain peace. When Kimberly and I both moved away and weren't forced to interact, we chose not to.

After I got married, John added a new dynamic to the family gatherings that took the focus off our sibling rivalry. Still, when I found out I was pregnant I wasn't sure what role, if any, Kimberly would play in our son's life. John and I don't have a large extended family, so I wanted Brady to have a relationship with his aunt. But considering the emotional distance between us, I wasn't hopeful.

Christmas Eve before Brady was born in February, I was surprised when Kimberly handed me a large, gift-wrapped box with a tag addressed to Brady. Yes, I had named my son shortly after the ultrasound. Once a planner, always a planner.

I opened the present and inside was a child's drum with two drumsticks attached by ropes. We all laughed at the gesture, which I took as a lighthearted message that she was going to encourage Brady to test my patience. And my hearing. But still, it was an olive branch, a recognition of her role as an aunt.

After Brady was born, Kimberly was tentative around him. She was not used to being around babies so it was understandable that she didn't want to hold him or play with him much in his infancy. But my dad, who had a special aunt in his life, encouraged her to do whatever she could to become a person of influence to Brady. And when Brady started to talk, everything started to change. Now that he could communicate with Kimberly and she with him, a new persona started to emerge that surprised us all. Auntie Kimberly was born.

Auntie Kimberly was not stoic, quiet, or serious. Auntie Kimberly was silly, funny, and willing to do whatever it took to make Brady happy. She wore crazy socks and ridiculous hats, and would show up at our door in costumes that catered to Brady's favorite things. She completely transformed in Brady's presence, and their bond grew quickly into one that is a driving force in Brady's life. And vice versa.

When Brady was diagnosed with autism, Kimberly jumped at the chance to help however she could. John and I would send out weekly newsletters to family, teachers, and therapists with updates on Brady's achievements, challenges, and learning objectives for the following week. Kimberly would create video content using a recurring cast of stuffed animals and digital characters to demonstrate the concepts. She would crank up the silly factor to the highest levels, but the message behind the fun was always impactful and hit its mark. Brady was hooked, and he would watch the videos over and over again.

When Kimberly was comfortable watching Brady alone, they started having playdates at her house that would last for hours. She had a stamina for entertaining him that I severely lacked, and the time she spent with him allowed me time to work, run errands, or even sneak in a nap.

Kimberly's impact reached far beyond therapeutic, however. She became the source of Brady's intense passion for all things *Star Wars.* When the series *The Mandalorian* premiered, she dubbed me the "Mommylorian" and documented on Facebook anytime I would try to curtail the number of sweet treats or extravagant gifts she would shower on Brady.

Auntie Kimberly promoted a love of "heavy metal" music, which thankfully was really just 1980s hair band rock. I got some serious "Mom cred" when Brady found out I'd not only heard of Guns n' Roses, but was in the front row for their concert in college. But Kimberly also loved classical music and helped Brady appreciate Mozart and Beethoven and Broadway musicals. They watched TV series and movies together, created YouTube videos of Brady unboxing toys and reviewing books, and even started their own band called T2 (short for the "Terrific Two").

Kimberly is also a talented writer, and created a series of fantastic tales called "Brady the Book Sailor." Brady was the main character who wielded a magical purple library card that could take him into the action of all his favorite stories. Brady the Book Sailor became a website that housed a collection of all of her creative poems, stories, and videos, and later showcased Brady's emerging artistic talents. They were two peas in a pod. They were perfect companions and best friends, and there was no doubt that Brady had filled an opening in Kimberly's heart that was exactly his size.

As Brady grew older, I worried he would start to outgrow their weekly playdates, but she easily transitioned their time together from playdates into hangouts. Their bond is stronger now than ever, and I am certain that nothing could ever come between them.

Kimberly's new role as Auntie Kimberly has had another effect; it brought us closer. Last summer we spent almost a week together with Brady, just the three of us. We talked and laughed about our childhood memories, played games, and ate junk food without having to ask permission.

When we said goodbye on the last day, I was sad that she was leaving. We stood there awkwardly until I finally took the plunge and leaned in for a hug. It obviously surprised her, because she coiled back slightly at first before she reciprocated by placing her arms lightly around my neck. It may have been the first embrace we'd shared in our entire lives.

I'm not sure a reconciliation would have happened with Kari and Kimberly. But with Mommylorian and Auntie Kimberly, anything is possible.

Sometimes God uses people around us to uncover who we are and who we are made to be. Through our relationships, dormant parts of our personality can come into the light and change us from the inside out. He gives us people in our lives who help us find our purpose, fulfill our purpose, and uncover our true identity.

Maybe you have a Gra inside you and can pour so much love on someone they feel like the most important person in the world.

Maybe you have a Dadat inside you and can love fiercely and encourage others who are different, like you.

Maybe you have an Auntie Kimberly inside you who is just waiting to bust out the silly socks so you can bring life and joy to someone who needs it.

Or maybe you can bring out the Gra, Dadat, or Auntie Kimberly in others. Remember, titles are important only if they reflect who God wants us to be. As W.C. Fields once said, "It ain't what they call you, it's what you answer to."

CHAPTER 20
THE LONG SWiM HOME

The Long Bridge Swim is a 1.76 mile open-water race in Lake Pend Oreille along the aptly named Long Bridge in Sandpoint, Idaho. When Brady was 12 years old he joined a swim team at the YMCA during the summer, and on the wall above the indoor pool was a sprawling mural of the event. It pictured hundreds of bodies in wetsuits, caps, and goggles descending into churned-up waters with nothing but the expanse of the lake in front of them. About a month before the event, Brady asked if he could participate, and simultaneously a small knot started to form in my stomach.

My knee-jerk reaction was no. Not because I didn't think he could finish the race. Brady had just spent an hour swimming in the lake with me paddleboarding alongside. He would have kept swimming even longer if I had let him, but I was the one who pooped out. No, my response was rooted in fear. My brain immediately started a ticker-tape list of all the things that could go wrong. Even so, somehow, I swallowed my outright rejection of the idea and said we could "look into it."

The FAQs on the website fanned my concern. The race results from prior years showed the winners were clocking in at about 35 minutes, but those in the bottom 20% had times of two hours or more. I knew Brady had a lot of stamina for swimming, but that was a long time for Brady to focus on something that didn't include a screen.

Second, he would have to board a bus at the local high school, which would take him to the starting line. Alone. No spectators or overprotective mamas allowed. The organizers suggested to worried parents they should register and swim with their kids, but I knew I could barely make it swimming 176 feet, much less almost two miles. How could I send him off with a bunch of strangers to accomplish a gargantuan feat without me?

If you are a parent, put yourself in my shoes. What would you have done? Let him register, or take the safe option of just laying down a firm parental "no"? I spent considerable time imagining what failure would look like for Brady. If he couldn't finish, or if he decided not to race at all, we might have to help him deal with shame, disappointment, and possibly even physical injuries. If we kept him from participating, he would be safe, but could miss an opportunity to conquer the biggest physical and mental trial of his life. These are decisions we all must wrestle with at some point—take the risk, or take the pass?

Ultimately, a free T-shirt and huckleberry ice cream at the finish line were no match for logic in the discussion with Brady, and we let him register.

Over the next several weeks there were a couple times when I thought he might drop out. If so, I would still get the credit for letting him sign up, but we would avoid the very real risks. Points without the pain, as my family used to say.

One day as he swam across the lake with me paddling nearby, Brady found himself in a pool of tiny fish skeletons—hundreds of them. I pretended not to notice, but I winced with each breath he took. I wanted to yell at him to keep his mouth closed, but I didn't want to alert him to the situation if he wasn't bothered by it. He kept on for another couple of minutes but finally started to give in to the creepiness of being surrounded by the masses of fish corpses. I thought I could displace the fish by having him swim behind the kayak, but nothing worked, and he frantically pulled himself into the boat. He was disappointed in himself for losing his composure, and I knew it was an opportunity for me to encourage him to quit, but I found myself doing the exact opposite. I pushed him to get back in the water.

The next few days of training were tough, because the little zombie minnows seemed to be floating everywhere Brady tried to swim. But after about a week he was past it, and the race was on.

In the meantime, the small knot in my stomach that had started when he registered grew into something that rivaled the world's biggest ball of twine. Which, in case you wondered, is housed in a "Ripley's Believe it or Not" museum in Branson, Missouri. I found myself counting down the hours until the whole thing was behind us.

Brady trained almost every day and showed incredible stamina in the water. He was making it through his two-hour swim practices with energy to spare, so my concern about the length of the swim started to subside.

Now, the source of my biggest fear was the bus ride. Even if Brady made it to the starting line without us, what if he realized the Herculean size of the challenge as the countdown began, and had an escape reflex? If he ran, how could we find him? He wouldn't have a phone, and he would disappear into the woods never to be seen again. I didn't tell Brady I was worried about the bus. First, I didn't want to create a self-fulfilling prophecy, and second, I didn't want to have the "When am I getting a phone?" conversation for the one-millionth time.

To make matters worse, the weather forecast was looking dicey. Lake Pend Oreille is a large, deep lake, the fifth deepest in the country. When the winds pick up the waves can resemble the wide-open ocean. Multiple weather services were predicting wind gusts up to 30 miles per hour the day of the race, which would mean treacherous conditions for the swimmers.

My only strategy was prayer. I prayed for God to calm the wind and waves, to be present with Brady, and to send angels to help us both get to the finish line. I was praying almost constantly as the race approached. If I wasn't talking out loud to someone else, I was praying quietly to God. I knew deep down that He was in control, but I won't lie and say prayer alleviated all my anxiety. Somehow my heart and brain were not explaining to my churning stomach that everything would be okay. But if you are facing something scary in your life, you have nothing to lose in giving it to God.

The night before the race John, Brady, and I all piled in the car to pick up Brady's registration packet. We showed up ten minutes early, but the high school lobby was already crowded with excited volunteers and swimmers. We found our "A-C" line, and chatted with a couple of veterans who assured me the event was safe and that I was not a terrible mother for allowing my twelve-year-old to go it alone.

When it was Brady's turn, he received a rubber swim cap that would be used to identify him, an ankle bracelet with an RFID chip that functioned as a timing mechanism, and a white trash bag that would hold his possessions. It was a combination of impressive technology and old-school simplicity. He wanted to put his favorite number, negative seven, on the cap and bag for good luck. I told him that would probably be confusing, since the registration number needed to go on the cap and bag. Fortunately, his registration number was 3327. The volunteer, overhearing our conversation, wrote the number seven extra-large with a line through it to represent the negative part. We were off to a good start.

We loaded up on thick-crust Hawaiian pizza for dinner since somewhere it is written that before a big athletic challenge you must stuff yourself with starchy, high-calorie junk food that basically negates the effort of the event before it ever happens. When it was time for bed, I knew sleep would be hard to come by, and not just because of the pizza baby that had formed in my digestive system.

After tossing around most of the night, I finally gave up and quietly slipped out of bed around 5:30 a.m. I walked out to the kitchen to start the coffee, and through our living room windows, I saw a single deer, only a few feet from our patio. It wasn't unusual to see deer in our neighborhood, but they were usually grazing at the far edges of the property, keeping lots of space between themselves and their human neighbors. But here she was, a beautiful doe looking back at me from just a stone's throw away.

I stood and stared at her for a full minute, and thanked God for giving me a visible sign of his presence, and an answer to my prayer. Just like the deer, sometimes God feels distant, but this morning He decided to remind me that He is always close.

Still gazing outside it dawned on me that I saw no movement in the small aspen tree leaves. I checked the weather on my phone and sure enough, there was no wind. The sky was gray with clouds and the temperatures were a bit cooler, but it was still. I couldn't see the lake from our home, but I prayed this wasn't a microclimate phenomenon. If not, the lake would be calm. Just like I asked, God calmed the wind and the waves.

When Brady woke up he could barely contain his excitement. He ate breakfast and wanted to put his wetsuit on right then, but we encouraged him to wait until a little closer to the race. I was relieved that John had devised a plan for communication as well. He had picked up a couple of walkie-talkies at a garage sale a few months earlier, and he placed one in Brady's white trash bag and one in our backpack in case Brady needed to reach us.

We set off for the safety briefing at the high school, and while I was comforted by the pieces of the puzzle falling into place, my digestive system still hadn't gotten the memo that everything was going to be fine. In just a few short minutes I was going to put my tween with autism and ADHD on a bus to face a huge challenge without me. I had almost tuned out the announcer by the time the buses started to arrive, but thankfully caught this very important tidbit—spectators could go on the buses as long as they waited for the swimmers to get on first. John and I would be able to go with Brady to the starting line!

I thanked God again and again. When I got on the bus with Brady, he asked if we could NOT talk about the race until we got to the starting line. I suppressed the urge to repeat the safety instructions again, and let him riff about the new *Loki* trailer, the next Batman movie he was going to watch, and the episode of the TV show *Psych* we watched the night before. We stopped talking completely when the bus started over the long bridge toward the starting line. We just held hands and I tried to visualize Brady in the water that was flying by below us.

When we got off the bus, the swimmers had to line up on a narrow path to the shore. This was where we had to say goodbye. I was grateful to see Brady this far, but I was still dreading letting go of his hand. John and I hugged him and told him how proud we were. Just then, a tall, older gentleman leaned into the conversation and pointed at Brady. He asked, "Is this his first time?" When we said it was, he introduced himself as Bart. He said his daughter swam her first race when she was twelve, and promised to take our son with him to start the race. There it was—God sent us an angel just like we asked. We left Brady with Bart and walked up to the bridge to watch the race.

It seemed like it took forever to see Brady emerge from the shoreline, but we eventually saw his green cap with his oversized negative seven streaming through the water. We were close enough that he could hear our voices, and he could talk back. We walked slowly across the Long Bridge keeping our eyes on him and encouraging him every few minutes. He never stopped, never held onto a kayak, or even rolled over on his back to float. He looked focused and determined, alternating between freestyle and breaststroke in rhythmic form.

When he finally emerged from the water an hour and a half later, he jogged sluggishly through the finish line. On the loudspeaker I heard a woman's voice proclaim, "Brady Baker just finished the race, and he's only twelve years old!" The crowd cheered. I cried as I hugged him tightly to my chest. My tears were fueled by his overwhelming achievement, and also relief that it was over, and he was safe.

It wasn't lost on John and me that the result could have been very different that day. All the alternate scenarios that stoked my fears over the last month could have happened. There have certainly been other trials Brady has faced in his life that didn't result in victory. But even during challenges where he didn't make it to the proverbial finish line, he learned something that got him to *this* finish line. As the great philosopher Yoda said, "The best teacher, failure is."

It's the same for you and me. Both personally, and as parents. As we face mountains that seem too steep to climb, we must remember that rewards rarely come without risk. It would have been much easier to keep Brady from entering the race. I would have saved a few gray hairs and valuable sleep knowing I wouldn't have to pick up the pieces if something went wrong. But now Brady has another memory planted in his soul that no one can take away. The next time he is faced with a test of his physical, mental, or spiritual strength, he will once again remember he can do hard things, and he will remember how to do it. With training, grit, perseverance, and lots of prayer.

After a double scoop of huckleberry ice cream and two glazed donuts we were back on the bus, and Brady was holding my hand. Just then a text came in from my dad, a private reply to my notice to family that he emerged from the lake unscathed. Dad had been on his own journey of faith and still had lots of doubts, but he told me that for the first time in fifty years, he prayed. He prayed for Brady's safety.

Brady and I exchanged tearful glances, and I squeezed his hand. This time we didn't talk about Batman. Brady told me how he prayed to God before the swim, and how he couldn't have finished the race without God. Neither could I.

CHAPTER 21
THE MAiN iNGREDiENT

I love garlic. I have been known to "accidentally" double the number of garlic cloves recommended for a recipe, and on occasion, I wind up spending the next day smelling like a villager in Transylvania terrified of a visit from Dracula. I also love salt. While I can usually control myself with most sweets, if you put a bag of salty crunchy snacks in front of me it is likely I will consume a full day's worth of calories in one sitting. So needless to say, garlic salt is one of my favorite seasonings and I use it in abundance when I need a quick hit of flavor in my recipes.

One night I mindlessly reached into the spice cabinet for my Costco-sized container of garlic salt when a strange thing happened—I couldn't lift it off the shelf. Confused, I kept tugging, but I was too short to see what was preventing me from accessing my powdered delight. Finally, the plastic jar came loose, and underneath it streamed thick lines of golden goo. I lifted to my tippy toes so I could get a better look and noticed a pool of the gummy substance covering the base of the cabinet. The pool led to a single stream up the left side of the cupboard and under the second shelf. I grabbed a footstool and climbed up to find an old, plastic, bear-shaped container of honey had mysteriously fallen and cracked open. Now half of my oils, spices, and other cooking accouterments were frozen in nature's super glue.

My heart sank as I realized that my big Friday night plan to work on my 1,000-piece puzzle was going to have to wait until I could free my seasonings and rescue my cabinet. I dreaded the process and had the thought that it might be easier to just rip the cabinet from the wall and get a new kitchen.

John helped me remove all the tainted bottles and jars from the cabinet. We placed everything on a large piece of packing paper and surveyed the damage. John suggested we could put a hairdryer on the honey, hoping the heat would loosen its grip on the plywood. I was skeptical and preferred the kitchen remodel idea.

I doubted we were the first homeowners to face this kind of mess, so I grabbed my phone and Googled "how to clean up spilled honey in a kitchen cabinet." Wouldn't you know it, the internet delivered step-by-step clean-up instructions.

The home hack website recommended boiling water, soaking a rag in the steaming hot water then laying it down over the honey. Supposedly the heat would extract the stickiness somehow and allow the honey to be wiped away. I guess my husband was on the right track with the hair dryer idea.

Incredulous but desperate, I got a pot, filled it with water, and within a couple of minutes it hit a rolling boil. I stood on the step stool so I could see the top of the shelf, and my husband fed me sheets of dripping, scalding towels until I completely covered the first pool of honey. I gave the rags just a second to cool so they wouldn't scorch my skin when I applied pressure to wipe the honey away, and to my surprise and relief, it worked! Within minutes our cabinet was clean.

I moved on to rescuing my spices by dipping them into the boiling water and easily wiping away the honey. It was a kitchen miracle, and I was able to settle into my Friday night puzzle after all. As a side note, it was also a good excuse to throw away the smoked paprika and cream of tartar that expired just before the turn of the century and to re-alphabetize my spice rack.

Isn't it interesting that sometimes the messiest situations in our life can be cleansed only by going through extreme, sometimes painful heat? Heat disinfects, it purifies, it takes something sticky and sets it free.

For years my life plan had been chugging along uninterrupted. Not to say there weren't bumps and hard times, but from a macro perspective, everything was working out. I found Mr. Right, albeit a little later in life than I'd hoped. We got married and bought a house. I had the child I always wanted, and then God threw me a curveball. Autism forced me to swerve onto a road I never wanted to visit. I kept turning back, trying to find a way back to the route I planned to take, but it was gone. Each step I took erased the ground behind me. I had no choice but to press forward.

What I finally came to realize is that the detour was not the problem. Even before autism, my recipe for a perfect life was missing the main ingredient. I was stuck. Underneath the surface of my visible façade, was an invisible anchor that was keeping me from moving toward true contentment, peace, and purpose. I had placed all my joy in the successful execution of my plan, instead of in the Author of my plan. When I was forced to abandon the life I thought I deserved, I felt the heat of disappointment, anger, and resentment. I had to hit a boiling point in order to break free.

God found me in the broken pieces of my prideful plan. For many Christians, it takes a crisis of control to reveal the overwhelming grace and goodness of our God. When we are on top of the mountain, we look down at the world below and believe our success is the result of our own planning and execution. When we tumble off the mountain into a valley, we are forced to look up for help. When we do, God is waiting with open arms full of peace that surpasses understanding.

If you haven't found your way to God yet, I pray that you don't have to endure suffering to get there. But if you do, remember that the fire you are walking through may be the cleansing you need to experience true freedom. He is preparing you for something new, equipping you to serve others, or softening your heart to welcome Him in. Just like in baptism—you enter the water a sticky mess and emerge a new creation.

Did you ever watch the TV Show, *Lost*? John and I started watching it after the first few seasons had already aired, and it was our first experience with "binge-watching." This was before Brady was born, so we could spend hours curled up on the couch without repercussions, except for extra pounds and sore backs.

The series starts with a plane crash on a remote island. There are dozens of survivors who, in *Lord of the Flies* style, have to learn to "live together or die alone." There are all kinds of surprises, mysteries, and dangers on the island, but as the characters fought for survival week after week, they not only overcame obstacles, but they evolved in the process. The doctor who was a control freak had to find faith and let go. The selfish conman bent on revenge became a hero who sacrificed himself for others. The fugitive from justice became a vigilant protector. The crippled man who was emotionally lost, found healing and purpose. But the most transformative catalyst to each character was not through the experiences they survived, but the relationships they formed with the other castaways.

Toward the end of the series, the protagonists are faced with a life-changing decision. They could go back in time and make it so that the plane never crashed. With a single action, they could return to the airplane, before the first bump of turbulence, and go back to life as if the crash never happened. I hate spoilers, so I won't tell you what they chose, but let me ask you. What would you do?

If you had the opportunity to turn back time, would you? If you had the power to snap your fingers and make it so that you never walked through your valley, never experienced the loss of a job or a relationship, never got that diagnosis, or never had to parent a special needs child, would you?

It's tempting, isn't it? I don't blame you if there is a part of you that would jump at the chance. On the surface you could avoid all the pain, all the sleepless nights, all the tears, and all the uncertainty that burdens you. I get it.

But in real life, we don't know what our story would look like without the tough chapters included. I would bet that even if you did get one free pass, one reset, one chance to set this trouble aside, your life still wouldn't be trouble free. You would have just replaced one hardship with another. Jesus tells us that in this life we will have trouble, so as much as we want to skip all the hard parts, we can't.

Just for argument's sake, let's say you could set aside your particular burden as if it never happened. What would you be giving up? Are there people you've met because of your challenge who have touched your heart? Are there skills you have been forced to acquire during your battle that may help you later in life? Did you gain perspective that was missing before, that has changed your worldview today? Is there someone out there going through a similar situation you are now in a position to help?

Simply stated, are you willing to give up who you are today, for who you were before? For me, the answer is simple. No way.

Autism was the hot water that I needed to set me free from my pride, independence, and control issues. Without autism, I wouldn't have returned to the one true God who loves me and has been chasing me my whole life. Without autism, I wouldn't have found lifelong friends. Without autism, I wouldn't have found joy in leading worship and a Bible study so I can help others find Jesus. Without autism, I wouldn't have a better relationship with my sister. Without autism, I wouldn't have experienced all the soul-stirring miracles of Brady's accomplishments.

Perhaps most importantly, without autism, Brady wouldn't be Brady. He is fearfully and wonderfully made. He is smart, funny, kind, truthful, faith-filled, and fearless. He is exactly the child I prayed for and more. He is a gift to me, and to the world. He was put on this planet for a purpose, so the world could see the works of God through him, just like John 9 promised.

Before I leave you, I want to share a revelation about John 9 that hit me as I was writing this book. If you remember, Jesus tells the disciples that neither the blind man nor his parents had sinned to cause his condition. Those verses changed my life and have been my inspiration ever since. But as Scripture tends to do, the Lord recently revealed something new to me in John 9. The words haven't changed, but my perspective has.

You see, I always pictured Brady in the role of the blind man and put myself in the position of the blind man's parents. After all, Brady was the one born with autism. I related the blind man's physical disability to Brady's neurological differences. But what if I had it backwards? What if I was the blind person?

Turns out, I was the one who needed healing and transformation. I needed to be cleansed and set free. I needed to know that I have a purpose on this earth beyond my selfish, controlling plan. My disability may not have been something that medical doctors could diagnose, but still, it impaired my capacity to live a love-filled, faith-filled, gratitude-filled life.

When my well-calculated plan fell apart, I did too. I needed to be pushed into the pot of boiling water to come out free from the things that made me blind. I was blind to all the blessings I should have been grateful for. I was blind to the miracles God was performing in my son. I was blind to the gifts God gave me to help others. And I was blind to the peace only God can give us when we are faced with a mountain we don't know how to climb. When my eyes were opened, when I could really see, I started learning to trust God to equip me for what is ahead, and to position me to bring glory to Him.

Coming to faith is not a ticket to life on easy street. I still have regular fits of impatience, frustration, and exhaustion. Autism still presents us with daily challenges, and even though I wouldn't change the past, sometimes I wish I could fast forward through the hard times. It's okay to feel that way in the moment, as long as you don't get stuck there.

So, if you are going through a valley today, here is my closing advice:

- Don't misinterpret your pain as punishment.
- Don't be blind to the gifts and growth you are picking up along the way.
- Don't ignore that you and your child were made on purpose, for a purpose.
- Don't forget who and *Whose* you are—you are God's beloved child, and He does not make mistakes.

- Don't go to sleep at night without gratitude for something, even if it is just the breath in your lungs.
- Don't assume that because your plan was derailed, that God doesn't have an even better one in mind.
- Don't give up hope that miracles can happen.
- Don't be stuck, be free.

Lastly, if you have been down a challenging path, remember to turn around and reach back for others. You don't need to provide answers or solutions, just time and attention. I will never forget those moms who stayed on the phone with me in the early days of our journey. They were my lifeline. This is your chance to be someone else's.

In the Bible, Paul writes in 2 Corinthians that God comforts us in our troubles, so that we may comfort others. You don't have to write a book or start a podcast. Just have a conversation, send a text, or pray. If you help one person, you are fulfilling God's wish. You have no idea how your encouragement may change the trajectory of someone's life.

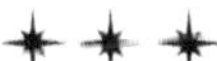

Our KIND story does not have a finite ending, and I'm done trying to plan one. I'm sure the next few years of living through puberty with a menopausal mother will create some spicy situations for Brady to overcome. But if I have anything to say about it, he will never doubt that his brain is the product of precise planning by the only Planner who matters. He will embrace his KIND-ness, claim his identity, and fulfill his purpose—so that God's works can be displayed in him. My prayer is the same for you.

ACKNOWLEDGMENTS

I never planned to have a child with autism. I never planned to write a book. I certainly never planned to write a book about raising an autistic child as a testimony of faith. But as I unpacked in the pages of *Finding KIND*, my plan was not God's plan. Thank goodness! God's plan is so much better. I can't even fathom all the variables that had to align and all the people who contributed to bring this book to fruition. Only God could pull it off. *Finding KIND* is not a reflection of my efforts, but His.

So first and foremost, thank you God for entrusting me to be Brady's mom, and for the gift of KIND Families. I pray this book reaches the hands and hearts of those who need it, while honoring You and Brady.

To **MOM AND DAD**–your transformation into Gra and Dadat has been my greatest joy to watch. My whole life you have loved me fiercely and supported me unwaveringly. Your commitment to Brady's happiness and development has been a critical factor in the wonderful young man he's become. I love you more than words can say.

To my sister **KIMBERLY**–thank you for being Brady's best friend and making him the center of your world. Your fingerprints are all over Brady's personality, sense of humor, and character. Everyone needs an Auntie Kimberly in their life.

To **GRANDMA SANDY**–you are the perfect complement to Brady's artistic, creative, and imaginative mind. Thank you for always freely sharing your faith and intense devotion with our family.

To all the **KIND MOMS** I've met over the last decade–you are all super mamas, and you inspire me every day. To **GINETTE** and **NEELY**, thank you for taking a call from a complete stranger and staying on the phone to quench my thirst for answers and direction. To **AMY** and **AMBER**, thank you for speaking my language and making me feel at home at a time when everything felt foreign. **DANA**, thank you for years of friendship inside and outside of autism and giving Brady a lifelong buddy.

To my great eight girls **LISA, CLAIRE** and **SARAH**–thank you for loving me, believing in me, and helping me believe in myself. You are the best cheering section a girl could hope for. Lisa, thank you for making me an "auntie" to Sydney and Riley, and giving Brady his first friends and closest "cousins." Your family is my family.

To **BOB GOFF** and **KIMBERLY STUART**–thank you for your wisdom and insight. Your enthusiasm and support kept me from jumping ship from this wild endeavor more than once! Bob, your book *Dream Big* was the spark that lit the fire for *Finding KIND,* and you are the reason *The KIND Families Podcast* exists. Kim, you could have doused the flame the first time we met, instead you fanned it. You are the writer I aspire to be; one with whom the reader laughs, cries, and wants to drink large amounts of sugary coffee. You are both the best KIND of people, those who love with abandon and share your talents generously. I am honored to have worked with you both and to count you as friends.

To everyone at **MCDOWELL CHURCH**–thank you for watering the mustard seed of my faith and helping it grow into a firm foundation for my life. **KYLEE KNAUSS**, your tangible love of Jesus at my first Bible Study made me want to love Him too. And

AGGIE THOMPSON, thank you for listening to the Holy Spirit and telling me to write a book, which seemed crazy at the time. Only God knew it would be a reality so many years later!

To my Revolution girls, **HEATHER**, **JAMEE**, **TAMY** and **TARA**–walking with you through life's mountains and valleys has provided scaffolding around my growing faith. Your friendship, love of Jesus and passion for following Him is an essential nutrient in my life. Tara, your God-given talent for design and generous heart brought KIND Families to life.

To **TEDI**, my unofficial spiritual director–your sweet friendship, wise counsel, and fervent prayer are gifts from God. You and Dick have rightly earned a position as Brady's honorary grandparents.

To the **THERAPISTS**, **DOCTORS**, **TEACHERS**, **AIDES**, and **FRIENDS** who helped our KIND family thrive–I am forever in your debt for the care and love you showered on Brady. I couldn't name them all over the last ten years, but a special thank you to **DR. RAUN MELMED**, **DR. JOE GENTRY**, and **MCKENZIE BOGARDUS MURPHY**. You changed Brady's life, and in turn my life, for the better.

To the **SOUTHWEST AUTISM RESEARCH & RESOURCE CENTER (SARRC)** and **PATTY DION**, founder of Think Asperger's–your outreach was the catalyst that started our KIND journey. Awareness is the prerequisite for early intervention, and you provided both.

To **EVERYONE AT BLUE HAT PUBLISHING**, especially **BRANDON JANOUS** and **RACHAEL MITCHELL**–thank you for your enthusiasm, guidance, and expertise throughout the editing and publishing process. Your integrity and thoughtfulness gave me peace of mind and confidence in the final product. I know our meeting was not by chance, and I'm grateful for your partnership and friendship.

Finally, to **JOHN AND BRADY,** my partners in KIND:

JOHN, you didn't have to let me chase this dream. Thank you for granting me the time and space to bring *Finding KIND* to the world, even though it meant putting some of your aspirations on hold. Publishing a book about our family is a delicate and vulnerable experience, one I know is difficult for you. I hope every reader grasps how wonderful you are as a husband and father. We are a great team and I love you and the life we've built.

Last but never least, **BRADY**, my sweet boy–thank you for helping me "find" KIND, and along with it my purpose and passion. You are so brave for letting me share our story to help other families. You are KIND in every aspect of the word. Never forget that you are fearfully and wonderfully made, and you were created exactly the way God intended to show His glory to others. I love you to the moon and back and even more than that, and more than anything in the whole wide world.

www.ingramcontent.com/pod-product-compliance
Lightning Source LLC
Chambersburg PA
CBHW031534260326
41914CB00032B/1793/J

* 9 7 8 1 9 6 2 6 7 4 1 4 0 *